Ophthalmology

For Churchill Livingstone

Publisher Mike Parkinson
Project Editor Dilys Jones
Copy Editor Sukie Hunter
Production Controllers Lesley W. Small, Debra Barrie
Sales Promotion Executive Duncan Jones

Ophthalmology

Hector Bryson Chawla

MBChB (St And) DO(Lond) DRCOG(Lond) FRCS(Edin) FCOphth
Consultant Ophthalmic Surgeon
Royal Infirmary, Edinburgh;
Examiner, Royal College of Surgeons, Edinburgh,
and College of Ophthalmologists

SECOND EDITION

CHURCHILL LIVINGSTONE
EDINBURGH LONDON MADRID MELBOURNE NEW YORK AND TOKYO 1993

CHURCHILL LIVINGSTONE
Medical Division of Longman Group UK Limited

Distributed in the United States of America by Churchill
Livingstone Inc., 650 Avenue of the Americas, New York,
N.Y. 10011, and by associated companies, branches and
representatives throughout the world.

First edition 1988
Second edition 1993

ISBN 0-443-04766-9

British Library Cataloguing in Publication Data
A catalogue record for this book is available from the British
Library.

Library of Congress Cataloging in Publication Data
A catalog record for this book is available from the Library of
Congress.

Produced by Longman Singapore Publishers Pte. Ltd.
Printed in Singapore

Contents

Preface

The seeds of this book took root from my total failure as a medical student to learn anything useful about the eye. However, over the years, I have discovered that the obstacle to learning is not the eye but ophthalmology. Somehow divorced from the mainstream of medical principles, ophthalmic tradition has never favoured a single sequence of examination, unchanging, no matter what might be wrong: instead we can make our choice from a whole collection of signs which we can then stretch to fit what we have guessed to be wrong.

Clearly, the diagnostic peaks are scaled only if we know the answer in advance, in which case, why bother to confirm what we have already decided? The approach falters if we do not know and comes to grief completely if, instead of the answer selected, we find another question or, worse still – two!

In times past, medicine was a meticulous description of the incomprehensible. Doctors prided themselves on a vast repertoire of observations, quaintly titled and invariably without rational foundation. Clinical acumen was measured by their ability to recognize, from an array of apparently identical observations, those patients who would recover from those who would not.

The sciences of physiology and pathology have gone a long way to put an end to all that, but sadly not in ophthalmology. In fact, the quagmire deepens with our determination to extend the choice of clinical features with a series of plus signs, with the result that where we once trod water, merely baffled, now we sink from view totally defeated.

Yet none of this needs to be. The eye is simply another part of the body. There is no reason why it cannot be examined in the same way every time as are the lungs or the heart or the legs.

There are only seven essential signs. They all relate to each other. The limited ocular response to disease can be described easily in permutations of the seven and not in a cloud of features expanding without check beyond the bounds of sanity.

Edinburgh, 1993   H. B. C.

ACKNOWLEDGEMENTS

My grateful thanks are due to my colleagues who have unstintingly contributed from their special areas of expertise;
  to Stuart Gairns for all the colour plates;
  to Ania Tokarcyk for her help with the illustrations;
  to Sandra McDonagh who never flinched when her final manuscripts turned out to be only drafts.

The following pharmaceutical companies helped in the production of this book:
  Alcon Laboratories
  Allergen Therapeutics
  Ciba Vision Ophthalmics
  Ethicon Ltd
  Leo Laboratories
  Vision Pharmaceutical.

1. A special organ made up of common tissues

The eye is a mobile sphere upon which the principles of a camera are based. A variable aperture regulates the amount of light entering; a transparent optical system focuses this light and a concave film picks it up.

It would seem that very special tissues are necessary to perform this marvel, but the elements of its construction are to be found in other parts of the body.

The outer coat of the globe (the sclera) is like the ball of a joint which moves in a socket of muscle, bone and eyelids. It is formed of collagen fibres and is heir to the same diseases that collagen can suffer elsewhere.

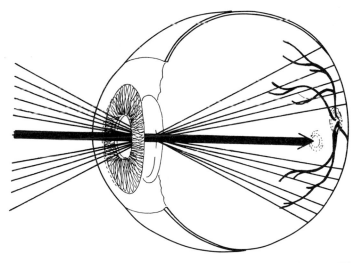

Fig. 1.1 A camera records what it sees without favour. The eye does not. The macular vision appears to dominate, but depends on a very tiny area of retina. The field of vision, occupying a much wider area of retina, gives matchless spatial information to people who do not even know of its existence.

A small segment of its anterior half – the cornea – differs from all the rest by being transparent. It begins the process of bending transmitted light.

The middle coat is a mixture of blood vessels, pigment cells and muscle, woven together by connective tissue. It is visible in front as the iris, where its dappled shades have given rise to much languid poetry and not a few rash decisions.

The hole in the centre of the iris is called the pupil. The pupil constricts to protect the retina when the surrounding illumination is too bright and dilates when it is not. The iris merges backwards into the ciliary body, which has three major roles:

1. as the source of aqueous fluid it is the very heart of the eye
2. its zonular ligaments hold the lens in place
3. its ciliary muscle is the muscle of focus.

At the ora serrata, the ciliary body gives way to the choroid, which is a sort of vascular undercoat between the sclera and the

Conjunctival sac

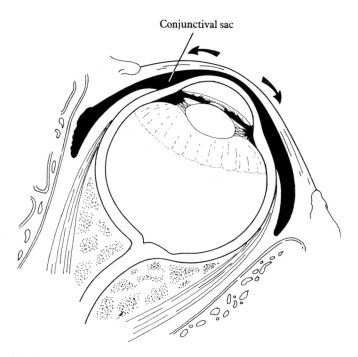

Fig. 1.2   The eye moves like a ball in its socket, lubricated by tear film and folds of conjunctival synovia. It can suffer from obscure rheumatic inflammations like other 'joints'.

pigment retina. Fed itself by the short ciliary arteries that cluster into the eye round the optic nerve, it feeds:

1. the disc
2. the pigment retina
3. the outer layers of the neuro-retina.

The classicists of pre-ophthalmoscopic days never saw a red reflex, but they did see a black reflex when the choroid or ciliary body bulged through a thin sclera or the iris actually prolapsed from a ruptured globe. Being epicures as well as classicists, they called the middle coat the uvea, from its fancied resemblance to the bloomed contours of a Burgundy grape.

The inner coat is the retina – a continuation forwards of the optic nerve – and both are part of the brain. Like all special tissues, the retina has reached such a pinnacle of refinement that it can never stoop to mere reproduction.

The retina actually consists of two quite separate layers:

— the outer pigment retina, which is firmly attached to the underlying choroid

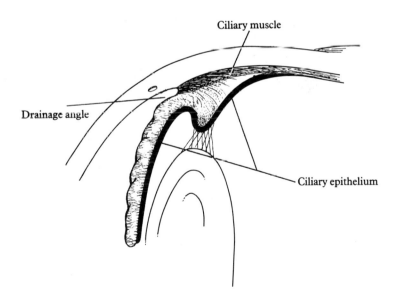

Fig. 1.3   The epithelium of the ciliary body, as the source of aqueous, is the very heart of the eye. The ciliary muscle alters the focus of the lens, which itself is slung from the ciliary processes.

— the inner neuro-retina, which is potentially separable from its fellows.

The two merge at the ora serrata, a critical landmark that corresponds to a line running around the eye through the insertions of the four rectus muscles. The fused pigment retina and neuro-retina continue forwards as the epithelium of the ciliary body and of the deep surface of the iris.

As might be guessed, the remaining ocular contents between the retina and the cornea are transparent.

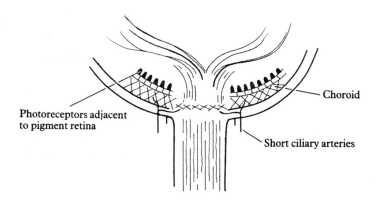

Fig. 1.4 The role of the choroid is to feed the optic nerve head, the pigment retina and the adjacent neuro-retina. The inner half of the neuro-retina – nearest to the vitreous – is supplied by the central retinal artery.

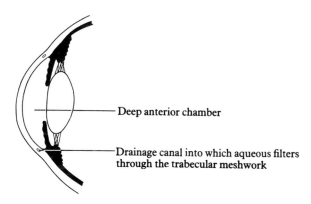

Fig. 1.5 The anterior chamber is that gap between the iris and the cornea. If it is deep, acute angle closure is impossible and one of those drugs marked 'Contraindication: glaucoma' can be used freely if indicated.

The anterior chamber behind the cornea and before the iris is filled with aqueous fluid.

The lens behind the iris is rather like the hub of a wheel spoked by the zonular ligaments to its rim, which is the ciliary body.

The remaining cavity behind the lens is filled with vitreous gel, sometimes referred to by the more droll term of vitreous humour. Rather like a clear jelly that has not quite set, it adheres to the ora serrata and to the optic nerve head.

Each eye is almost totally surrounded by the bony walls of the orbit. Bone all the way round would certainly guard the eye, but visually the arrangement would be rather pointless. The eyelids take over where the bone ends. They open to allow the eye to see and close to protect it. Their shape is maintained by a fibrous plate. They are moved by muscles and they are allowed to move by the concertina qualities of their superficial and deep surfaces.

The outer layer is skin, adherent to the plate and thrown by the opened lids into the folds at the orbital margin, where the lid skin merges with the facial skin.

The inner layer is a synovial membrane, which is also adherent to the lid. It blends eventually with the corneal epithelium and its loose folds take the form of an apple-pie bed that encircles the globe behind the equator.

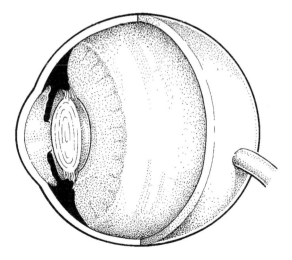

Fig. 1.6 The lens is the hub of the ciliary wheel. The rim is the ciliary body and the spokes are the ciliary processes and the zonular ligaments.

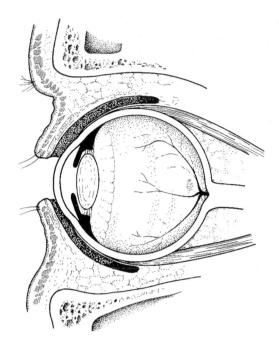

Fig. 1.7   The eye is surrounded by the bony orbit, except in front, where the protective eyelids have to open some of the time if the eye is to be more than just a precious organ to be guarded but not used.

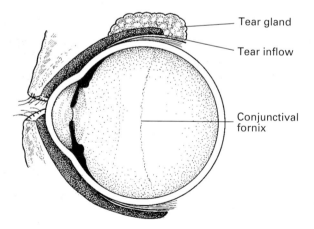

Fig. 1.8   The conjunctiva is a member of the external quadruple alliance. Its upper fornix and lower fornix spread loosely around the globe, like the fold of a circular apple-pie bed. (The increasing popularity of eiderdown quilts is making the apple-pie bed a historical curiosity.) The tear gland is another member of the alliance, its secretions helping the lids to give the eye, when open, the comfort it enjoys when closed.

Both the conjunctiva and the cornea are kept moist by the lacrimal gland, which is neatly placed above the lateral aspect of the eye to duct its tears into the upper fornix of the conjunctival sac.

Although well known as manifestations of sorrow, emotion, frustration and blackmail, tears have a more prosaic and vastly more important function as lubricant and blood substitute for the cornea.

They are not just bitter salt as the poets would have us believe. They also contain both lipid and mucus, which increase the wetting effect of the aqueous component and delay evaporation.

Any remaining tears drain away through little holes in the eyelids called puncta and along minute canals to collect in a tear sac, whence they flow along yet another duct into the nose. The macroscopic and microscopic arrangement, and indeed their general behaviour, are not unlike that of the ureters, bladder and urethra.

The last structure on the outside, the eyelashes, are hair 'by any other name'. Their cat whisker sensitivity, which triggers the blink reflex, is invariably ignored by their owner when she is bent on adorning the lids with seductive pigments.

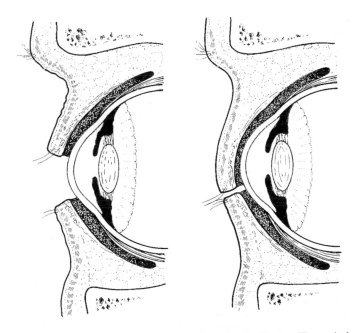

Fig. 1.9   The eyelids are part of the external quadruple alliance. The eyelashes are the 'cat's whiskers' which trigger the blink reflex.

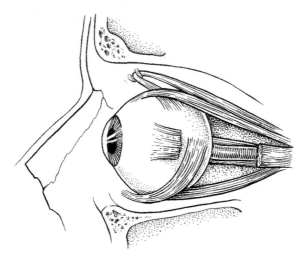

Fig. 1.10 Four rectus muscles and two oblique muscles move the eye in any direction in concert with its fellow.

If the whole point of the eye is to see, the whole point of both eyes is to see together. Six muscles move each eye under instruction from the motor cortex and from the lower centres. There are of course two eyes and each gazes upon the world from a different viewpoint. The brain fuses these two separate flat views into one single view in depth. This three-dimensional faculty is called binocular vision.

The remaining space in the orbital cavity is filled with arteries, veins, cranial nerves and fat.

It must be plain that the organ of mystery is just another collection of familiar tissues – curious perhaps in its shape, worrying in the sum of its parts, but totally commonplace when each part is taken in isolation.

THE TRANSPARENT TISSUES

The one unique quality of the eye is that it is partially transparent. Like any other optical system it is fashioned from a series of focusing structures which are clear and held together by a series of supporting structures which are not.

Unlike other optical systems, the eye is composed of living tissues and all such tissues require a feeding and waste disposal system. The opaque elements can make do with blood, which is also opaque, but the transparent elements cannot. They need something that is also transparent. This role is taken on by the aqueous fluid.

The transparent components are:

— the cornea
— the anterior chamber
— the aqueous
— the lens
— the vitreous.

The retinal layers nearest the vitreous are also light permeable because the photoreceptors have to lie in contact with the pigment retina.

The cornea

This anterior window into the eye transmits and focuses light. Its health first of all depends on snugly fitting eyelids. It could not remain moist and clear and safe from injury without being covered, and obviously it would be useless to the eye unless it could be uncovered. The lids blink reflexively to remove unwanted foreign bodies and to coat the corneal surface with a smooth film of tears, making it glisten as any quality refracting surface should.

Anything that separates the contact between the lids and the cornea – for example, a facial palsy – puts the smooth surface in danger of replacement by scar tissue. This does very well as a protection but less well as a transmitter of light.

Because the cornea is the one clear structure that presents a surface to the external world, it cannot rely on aqueous alone. The aqueous supplies the deep layers, but the superficial layers have to depend on tears.

There are no sharp edges in nature and scleral blood vessels occasionally loop over the corneal margin.

That is as far as they should go in health, but when a damaged cornea demands more of the tears and the aqueous than they can provide, these vessels may grow in to do their bit and, in so doing, ruin the cornea as a transparent structure.

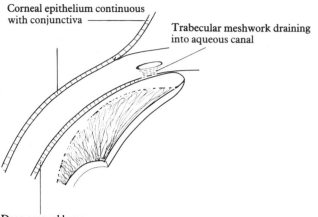

Corneal epithelium continuous with conjunctiva

Trabecular meshwork draining into aqueous canal

Deep corneal layer

Fig. 1.11   There are five corneal layers. The epithelium takes its oxygen from the tears. Penetration of the second layer disrupts the regular stroma into a scar. The deep layer keeps the cornea in a state of part-hydration.

The corneal stroma

As the forward continuation of the sclera, the cornea plays a part in maintaining the spherical shape of the eyeball and in protecting its contents. Its collagen fibres, though no different from those of the sclera in form, are rather different in their arrangement.

This actual arrangement has taxed the ingenuity of researchers, who have still not convincingly explained how the cornea allows a free passage of light. It is suggested that the fibres lie in a two-dimensional lattice just less than a wave-length of light apart. By some subtle mechanism the visible spectrum passes through, where in some other arrangement it might not.

Such a hypothesis is certainly borne out clinically by the formation of scars – as opaque as any part of the sclera – that follows interference with the corneal stroma.

Two membranes mark the limits of the cornea. Its anterior surface is separated from its anterior epithelial layer by Bowman's membrane, penetration of which will always end in loss of stromal clarity.

Its deep surface is lined by Descemet's membrane, which separates the stroma from the cellular endothelial layer – deeper still.

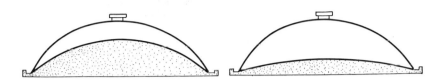

Fig. 1.12   The anterior chamber is like a serving dish and lid. The iris is the base and the cornea the lid. The more convex the base the more shallow the anterior chamber; the flatter the base the deeper.

The endothelial layer plays a vital part in the maintenance of clarity. It continually withdraws water from the corneal stroma, keeping it in a state of semi-hydration. Malfunction of this water pump has but one sequel – corneal oedema.

The anterior chamber

A certain mystery seems to shadow this space, which figures endlessly in discussion about other parts of the eye but somehow never seems to merit a word or two on its own account.

It is the aqueous filled gap, bounded in front by the cornea and behind by the iris–lens diaphragm. It fills with aqueous diffusing from the ciliary body. The chamber is not, however, stagnant; fresh aqueous enters through the pupil and old aqueous leaves through the trabecular meshwork.

It might be useful to imagine the chamber as a serving dish, with a transparent lid – the cornea, convex on its outer surface, concave on its inner surface and sitting against a gently convex base – the iris.

The depth of this anterior chamber varies with the convexity of the iris. When it is deep the iris is almost flat. When it is shallow, the convex iris almost touches the back of the cornea.

The lens

The lens is the hub of the ciliary body wheel. Although shaped like a lentil, as its name suggests, it is constructed more like a

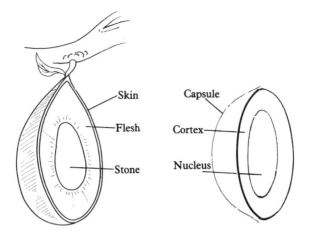

Fig. 1.13 The lens is like a transparent plum. The skin is the capsule. The flesh is the cortex. The stone is the nucleus. A plum when too ripe can burst and leak; so too can a lens, provoking a severe iritis and a grossly raised intraocular pressure.

transparent plum (without the stalk). The nucleus corresponds to the plum stone, the cortex to the flesh and the capsule to the skin.

The lens not only transmits and focuses light, it can also vary that focus. Variation is brought about by the ciliary muscle. This muscle maintains in age the power it had in youth, but as the years go by even this power is not enough to modify the shape of the hardening lens (presbyopia). It is for this reason that people lose the ability to make out near objects in their mid-forties.

The blood substitute of the lens is the aqueous. Any insult, whether it be an alteration in the composition of the aqueous or damage to the lens capsule, brings with it the risk of clouding. Whatever the cause, this loss of transparency is called cataract, but preferably not within earshot of patients, who all go in mortal dread of the name.

The vitreous

This is possibly the most inert tissue of the body, making the standard tendon appear almost lively by comparison. A whorl of fine collagenous fibrils separated by a gel of hyaluronic acid, it fills the cavity of the eye behind the lens. Its attachments in health are to the optic nerve and the ora serrata. The aqueous fluid drifting

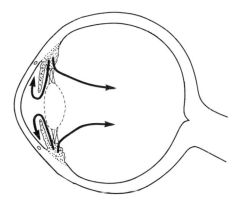

Fig. 1.14   Obvious disturbance to the outer eye can produce less obvious disturbance to the inner eye. Whatever happens to the eye, 'think aqueous'.

through serves its languid metabolic function. Any opacities resulting from disease clear away with equal languor, if they do so at all.

The aqueous

Without aqueous there would be no eye and without a grasp of its behaviour there can be no rational grasp of why the eye behaves as it does. It is so simple that everybody imagines that there has to be a catch somewhere.

Aqueous differs from blood in two ways:

1. it is clear
2. it does not circulate as part of a fixed volume system.

Aqueous is constantly secreted into the eye by the ciliary epithelium and just as constantly excreted through this trabecular meshwork in the angle of the anterior chamber.

Between entry and exit, it percolates throughout the eye feeding the transparent tissues, then it flows through the pupil to fill the anterior chamber.

The trabecular meshwork is rather like a circular sieve through which the major portion of the aqueous filters out of the aqueous chamber into the episcleral veins.

The aqueous not only feeds the transparent structures, it also maintains the shape and pressure of the eyeball and in health

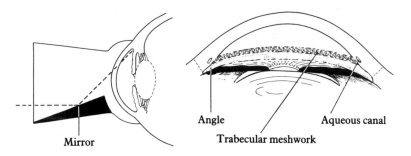

Fig. 1.15   Detail in the drainage angle is visible through a mirror set in a gonioscopy lens. In this open angle the trabecular meshwork is readily visible. In a closed angle it is not. *Gonia*, the Greek word for angle, explains the curious name.

there is a nice balance between what is produced by the ciliary epithelium and what flows out through the trabecular sieve. When that balance is upset, things begin to go wrong.

At one end of the scale, gross damage to the eye can wreck the ciliary body. The eye starving of aqueous becomes softer and softer until it can no longer maintain any resemblance to a round ball. The iris disappears behind a clouded cornea and the whole eye shrinks back into the orbit, the eyelids flattening as they follow the eye inwards. The term phthisis, culled from the nineteenth-century world of consumption, carries in its very syllables the sound of shrinkage, ruin and irresistible decline.

Lesser insults like surgery of one sort or another can stun the ciliary body and the eye may soften dramatically until the ciliary epithelium returns to full production.

At the other end of the scale, obstruction to the passage of aqueous through the pupil and out of the eye brings about the opposite. The eyeball hardens. And if aqueous cannot get out of the eye at the front, blood has equal difficulty in getting into the eye at the back.

Recent work has suggested direct damage to the optic nerve by the pressure itself, compounded by local ischaemia. In simplistic terms we may imagine the blood supply to the optic nerve squeezed to extinction and the visual field equally squeezed to extinction. The erosion of vision is not always noticed because it begins as islands of reduced sensitivity. The eyes succumb at different rates and the central vision succumbs last of all.

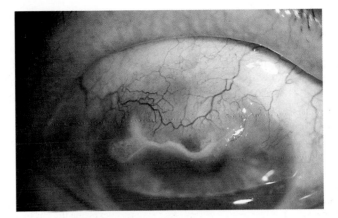

Fig. 1.16 Excavation at the corneal margin – many causes can produce an end result like this. The blood vessels have infiltrated an area normally avascular because disease has increased its metabolic needs beyond those supplied by tears.

We call this process 'glaucoma'. If a cause be known we can call it glaucoma secondary to that cause. When no cause is known, we slip into that comfortable medical jargon of fluent ignorance that passes for knowledge, and call it glaucoma simplex.

The epithelium of the ciliary body is therefore the heart of the eye. The behaviour of the aqueous it produces lies at the very heart of understanding how the eye behaves in health and in sickness.

SUMMARY

It must now be evident that the eye and its supporting structures have infinitely more in common with the rest of the body than is usually supposed. All but three of the tissues are duplicated elsewhere. These three tissues share transparency as their common factor.

They achieve this quality by their internal arrangement, their shape and their dependence on blood substitutes. When defeated by any disease process, they are prepared to exchange their unique privileges in return for simple survival. Where once they played a patrician role, bathed in tears or aqueous, they descend to accept the infiltration of blood vessels rather than die. The price they pay is the loss of their special qualities. They are rather like a putting surface taken over by weeds – acceptable as grass but not as the 18th green at Augusta National.

As for the aqueous, it is perhaps the most misunderstood of all the intraocular contents. It does not circulate, it flows from the ciliary body to the trabecular meshwork. Balance of inflow and outflow must be just right. Too much aqueous can destroy the field. Too little aqueous can destroy the eye.

To 'think aqueous' is to understand the eye. From there it is but a step to translate that understanding into a rational foundation of diagnosis and management.

2. How the eye sees

NORMAL VISION

The eye possesses two quite different faculties – central vision and field vision. Although they are both served by the same retina they are quite separate in position and quite different in function.

Whilst it is customary to compare the eye with a wide-angled camera, there are two well-defined dissimilarities.

First of all, the camera film is flat, whereas in the eye it is cupped, rather like a brandy goblet. Secondly the camera does not discriminate what it records: detail is equal throughout. The eye, on the other hand, picks out one object to fix on, whilst recogniz-

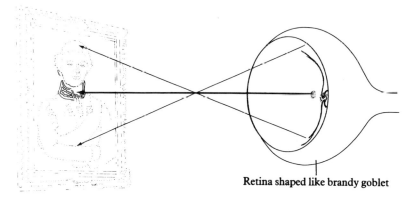

Retina shaped like brandy goblet

Fig. 2.1 Foveal detail may appear to dominate the vision, but objects in the field, like brush strokes on a canvas, add character and the very essential background against which to appreciate what the macula happens to be concentrating on. The macula, scanning constantly, creates the illusion that all vision is detailed and it is for this reason that attempts to capture landscapes and impressions with a camera are usually so disappointing.

ing the presence of others, and recognizing less of them the further they lie from the centre of fixation.

Although it might seem to us that our central vision merges imperceptibly into our field vision, there is no such gentle gradation in the retina.

The central retina is dominated by the macula; it is quite possible to lose the centre and keep the field. It is equally possible and visually far more devastating to do the opposite.

CENTRAL VISION

When the eye gazes at something, it is looking through the pupil along its visual axis. At one end of the visual axis is the observed object; at the other, in the depths of the 'retinal brandy goblet', is the macula.

The macula – the special area of central vision, compared with the rest of the retina, is tiny – some 5.5 mm across (the optic nerve head, the fundal yardstick, measures 1.5 mm). At the macular centre lies the fovea, which is the extra special area of the macula and is even more tiny still, measuring fractions of a millimetre.

Its precise refinement and colour sense depend on the macular photo-receptors – the cones which congregate here in large numbers and which function best in high illumination. Upon these cones is based that distinction between almost similar details, which is the essence of sharp visual acuity.

Just how sharp must be judged by trying to read adjacent words on a page of print, whilst maintaining fixation on one of them.

It is the one kind of vision that everyone knows about and because of its easy dominance, they do not realize that there is another. That smooth glide from central vision into field vision fools them into thinking that vision is all of a piece. It is not, and they are fooled at their peril.

FIELD VISION

Whilst disturbance of the central vision of either eye will produce a stream of patients wondering if the time has come to discard their grandmother's glasses, field loss in one eye raises no questions about glasses at all. But this field sense, served by the huge area of extramacular retina, is as important as it is self-effacing.

The peripheral retina contains both cones and rods. The cones operate during normal illumination. Rods, although useless for the recognition of colour, come into their own with increased sensitivity when illumination is reduced.

The field has been compared to an assortment of patterns but none of them conveys the perception that the size of the field is directly proportional to the distance from the eye at which we pick it up.

The field of each eye sprays forwards like a discharge of buckshot from an asymmetrical blunderbuss, the cone of vision widening without limit to infinity:

— on the temporal side – directly outwards – even backwards
— on the nasal side – at an angle crossing the line spraying from the other barrel.
— it also sprays upwards and downwards.

We can pick up its edges:

— 5 cm from the lateral orbital margin.
— 5 cm in front of the fellow eye
— 5 cm from the chin
— 5 cm from the junction of the forehead with the scalp.

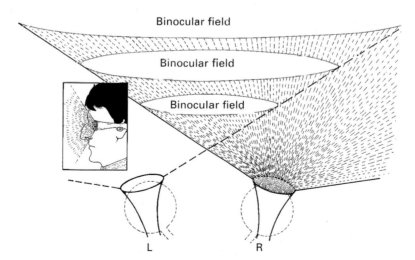

Fig. 2.2   The visual field from each eye is like a spray of buckshot from a blunderbuss.

The circular centre covered by the spray of vision from both eyes is called the binocular field.

Each eye retains a degree of independence, for the temporal spray provides a crescent of vision that belongs to that eye alone. This crescent at the temporal periphery can be demonstrated when fixation is maintained with the central vision on some immobile distant object and each eye is covered alternately.

Although the binocular field confers great advantages in perception of depth, the surviving field in one eye can mask the vanishing field in the other, and the patient may not realize that it is going until it is gone.

With an intact pathway running from the macula to the occipital cortex, it would be reasonable to imagine that normal central vision would exist automatically. Unfortunately an intact pathway is not enough, for central vision is not a birthright.

Macular stimulation is required to trigger development and sometimes the macula is not stimulated as well as it might be, nor as early.

There is some question about what is early enough, and the answer must vary with the extent of the deprivation. A congenital cataract, dense at birth, will totally deprive the eye of visual stimulation whilst an intermittent squint, 2 years after birth, sometimes reduces the visual stimulation and sometimes does not. Clearly the entire visual cortex can suffer from sensory deprivation but it is the macular loss which dominates.

An opaque congenital cataract therefore requires removal as soon as is technically possible. A less opaque one, with some evidence of visual function, might be left in place.

In general, anything that interferes with visual stimulation in early life will arrest development. It need not be a serious disease. It could be something as simple as an error of refraction that is greater in one eye than in the other and to which the body will respond by favouring the easy eye at the expense of the other.

We would probably have a diminishing opportunity up to the age of 5 years to persuade central vision to develop. In the case of total deprivation, 5 months is probably too late. In cases of discrepant refractive errors, successful intervention might still be commenced in the early teens.

The peripheral retina collects rough impressions of our surroundings that become less rough the nearer these impressions approach the sensitive macula. Because the macula is so sensitive, the rest of the retina is frequently considered by the partially informed as an extension of the macula and by the ill-informed not considered at all.

A patient reassured that all is well because of perfect central vision in each eye could already be losing visual field in both eyes. Perfect central vision certainly indicates that the macula and the relevant parts of the visual pathway are intact. It does not guarantee the integrity of everything else.

Visual testing is not complete unless it includes some rough estimate of the field of vision.

THE RETINA

This first appears in the embryo as a small balloon on a stalk derived from the forebrain. The anterior half dimples, then dimples a little more before sinking into the cavity of the balloon, where it forms two layers. The inner layer becomes the neuro-retina. The outer layer becomes the pigment retina. The layers unite at the ora serrata, which marks the anterior limit of the retina and the posterior limit of the ciliary body.

As part of the brain, the neural retina has an enormously com-plicated arrangement. However, its complications can be reduced

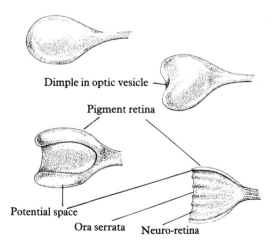

Fig. 2.3   There are two retinae. The outer pigment retina and the inner neural retina, attached at the anterior edge and at the optic nerve head, are potentially separable everywhere else. If fluid infiltrates this space the neuro-retina has detached.

to light receptors adjacent to the pigment retina, which then connect through a series of cells, finally ending as the nerve fibres of the innermost retinal layer. These fibres sweep from all areas of the retina, leaving the eye through the optic nerve head, of which synonyms are the optic disc or the papilla.

The light receptors contain an aldehyde of vitamin A linked with a protein molecule, and it is the realignment of these molecules in response to light that gives rise to visual perception. Although it might be impertinent to suggest that the arrangement could be better, it is worth comment that the retina overlying the light receptors has to be transparent, else the whole mechanism would be pointless.

Cones

Cone receptors abound in the macula where, as well as providing the visual precision of the central retina, they also distinguish one colour from another. They are also found in the peripheral retina where they provide a sense of form and colour in standard illumination.

Rods

The dominant receptors in the peripheral retina, they come into their own when reduced illumination has deprived the cones of their traditional dominance. This process is known as dark adaptation. It is lost in some retinal diseases, the most famous of which is retinitis pigmentosa.

The dark-adapted retina, dependent on rods, cannot recognize colour, and it is this feature which gives rise to that subtle yet heightened perception by moonlight – those honeyed shadows that daylight sharpens with an unpalatable edge.

The retinal blood supply derives from two sources. The choroid supplies the pigment retina and adjacent half of the neuro-retina. The central retinal artery, entering the eye through the optic nerve head, supplies the other half of the neuro-retina adjacent to the vitreous.

As part of the brain, the retina must have a copious blood supply. It will come as no surprise that the macular area, being the most subtle, is the one that suffers most when its blood supply is compromised.

The faltering blood flow of later years becomes more obvious at the macula than anywhere else in the retina. A retinal detachment involving the macula, no matter how briefly, even when successfully repaired, will usually leave its mark on macular function.

Focusing mechanisms

So far we have dealt with light entering the eye but no mention has been made of how this light is directed to the relevant parts of the retina from various distances. The optical diagrams that crop up in textbooks, just when ophthalmology is beginning to seem pleasant, have sadly persuaded many that the whole subject is just ophthalmo-babble, now totally ruined by unhappy memories of natural philosophy.

The terms long sight and short sight, which actually mean the opposite of what they say, start the ball of confusion rolling. Medicine abounds with confident mis-statements but none so confidently mis-stated as these. As with so much else in ophthalmology acquisition of the magic words endows them in the end with an existence quite separate from their alleged meaning.

Anyone who has set fire to paper with sunlight focused through a convex lens is already familiar with the principle of bringing light to a focus from infinity. The optical convention is that such light is drawn with parallel rays. The stronger the lens, the nearer its focal point will be to its surface.

Normal sight

Such an eye brings parallel rays of light to a focus from infinity without effort. Its ciliary muscle is relaxed.

Anything further away than 6 mm is considered to be at infinity.

For that reason, normal distance visual acuity is recorded at 6/6 (20/20 feet). The upper figure is the distance at which the test card is carried out. The lower figure is the distance at which the letter size ought to be seen.

6/12 means that the eye in question can make out only at 6 metres a letter which it ought to make out at 12 metres.

The normal eye can shift its focus from infinity to near. Just how near diminishes with age but most children, with chastening

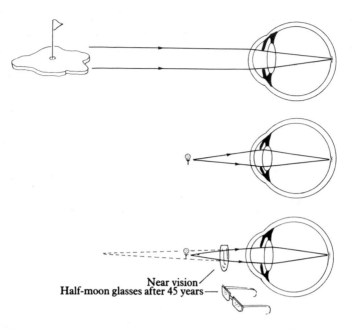

Fig. 2.4 The normally-sighted eye sees distant detail without effort. Up to the mid-forties it can, without effort, make out near detail as well. After the mid-forties, effort alone is not enough. Near vision glasses are required.

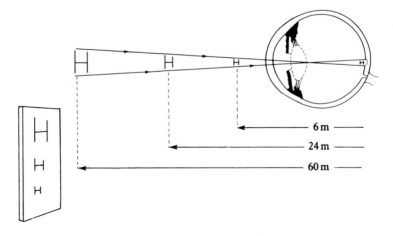

Fig. 2.5 The 6 m letter at 6 m and the 60 m letter at 60 m appear the same to the eye. The nearer the larger one approaches to the eye the bigger it will appear, because it throws an angle of increasing size at the macula. A magnifying glass magnifies because it allows things to be seen nearer to the eye than the eye can normally manage on its own.

skill, can discern detail at a couple of inches from the eye. The ciliary muscle contracts and the elastic tension on its capsule steepens its surface into greater convexity. The lens becomes fatter and more powerful and shortens its focal length.

The reading position chosen by most people is a product of habit and of arm length. Any test of near vision merely records the ability of the eye to make out print of decreasing size. As the years go by, the lens hardens and fails to respond to the directions from the ciliary muscle. This process begins in the early twenties but becomes recognizable only in the mid-forties when newspapers are not printed as well as they used to be and arms are suddenly found to be too short for comfortable reading.

Presbyopia is the name given to this humbling infirmity. It increases with age and lenses of increasing strength are required to compensate for the lost range of focus of the natural lens.

Long sight

When people talk of long sight they think they mean normal sight and they imagine marvels of distance vision. In truth, a really

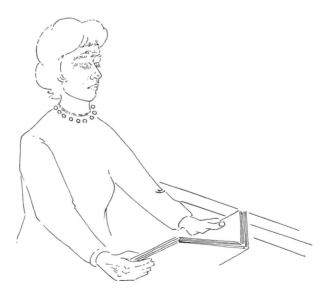

Fig. 2.6 Presbyopia – the denied evidence of passing time. Print is not what it used to be. The arms are becoming too short.

marked degree of long sight can actually prevent any effective vision whatsoever. Patients after cataract extraction without a lens implant have no doubt at all what long sight means.

The long-sighted eye has a focal length that is longer than the eye itself. The relaxed focal point would therefore lie behind the retina, were light able to pass through the back of the eye. The eye naturally wants to focus to the macula and sets the ciliary muscle to work to make this possible. The long-sighted eye may see in the distance but uses up its reading focus to do so.

Such an eye with all its focusing range exhausted finds itself unable to focus for near. Thus a 30-year-old with long sight could well find reading impossible. A lens to correct the distance vision will then release the normal range of focus of that age group to allow clear vision at the common reading distance.

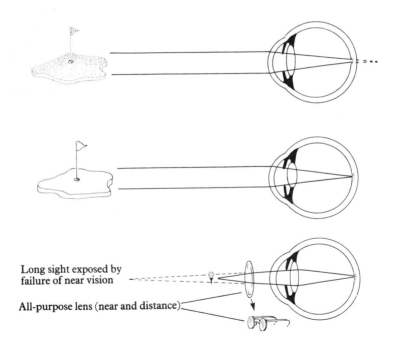

Long sight exposed by
failure of near vision

All-purpose lens (near and distance)

Fig. 2.7   The long-sighted eye sees distant detail without effort and has to use up its near focus to do so. It may have none left for near use even in the young. Up to the mid-forties the same correcting lens can be used for both distance and near vision. After the mid-forties something has to be added to the distance correction for near focus.

Short sight

Short sight means many things to many people, and most of them wrong.

The focus of such an eye is too short for the eyeball. Parallel rays of light from the distance come to a focus between the lens and the retina, sometimes giving a blurred hint of things of interest and sometimes not even that.

The object in view, therefore, has to be brought closer to the eyeball so that the rays of light diverging from it will push the focal point near enough the retina to be of use. Such eyes see near objects without effort, but pay the price of seeing little in the distance no matter what the effort.

It has been averred that such limitations influence the character of short-sighted people, making them bookish, withdrawn and unaggressive. It is not easy to strike a martial posture when one cannot actually see where to strike it. However, some dauntless myopes, spurning spectacles, have gone to war, seeing barely beyond their tent flaps. They accepted with some insight that their failure to see either army would have no influence on the course of the campaign; none was more dauntless or more myopic than Sir George Brown – one of the Crimean High Command.

He pointed his sword at what he thought was the enemy then launched his brigade through an adjacent column of his own

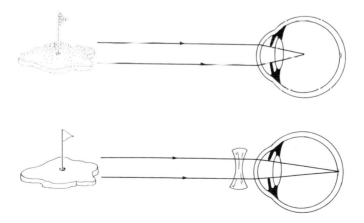

Fig. 2.8   The short-sighted eye cannot see in the distance, with or without effort. The eyelids can with effort close to a slit, which approximates to a pinhole in the middle at the price of crows' feet tramping over the skin where it is most visible.

army. The Russians, gazing in wonder at this advancing rabble, lost their nerve before what they took to be a new and irresistible military formation.

Astigmatism

All the foregoing refractive errors, as they are called, assume that the eye is a perfect sphere. Occasionally it is not, and sometimes the actual lens within the eye does not act equally in all meridians. It might be helpful to imagine such an eye as shaped like a rugby ball. It can never produce a point of focus either on the retina or off. If one meridian is sharp then the other by definition must be blunt and the resultant oval focus can never come to a point. The answer is an oval lens (cylindrical) focusing on one meridian only, and the eye will become optically spherical again.

MANAGEMENT OF REFRACTIVE ERRORS

The simplest way to deal with the optically deficient eye is to ignore the deficiency and pretend that the second-rate vision is in fact normal. This approach is more common than might be imagined.

Spectacles and contact lenses in all their variations are already very familiar. But the surgeon's approach to most things is to produce a scalpel and, at the extremes of visual inadequacy, several surgical approaches have been devised.

Contact lenses

Contact lenses are foreign bodies applied to the cornea in the hope that visual betterment or emotional relief from discarding spectacles will compensate for the insult to the eye of their application. Made from a variety of synthetic transparent materials of differing physical attributes, they are accepted by the eye only in the presence of a normal fluid exchange across the corneal surface and an adequate supply of tears.

These conditions are not always met. Fluid balance throughout the body fluctuates as the normal hormonal cycles fluctuate, and when these cycles are further unbalanced by the contraceptive pill, pregnancy or impending abortion, intolerance of contact lenses may be the first indication. Should the tear secretion decline below a certain critical level, then this intolerance becomes permanent.

Even healthy eyes have their problems. Coarsely fitted lenses depriving the anterior corneal surface of oxygen will cause a hazy oedema of the epithelium. Over-wearing of well-fitted lenses will produce the same result, and if carried to foolish lengths may induce the growth of superficial new vessels around the corneo-sclereal limbus – presumably to make up the oxygen normally supplied by the tears.

With this baleful array of hazards it is a wonder that people wear contact lenses at all. They do so for a variety of reasons. Vanity and cosmetic satisfaction can lead to a tolerance of the most appalling discomforts, and most contact lenses are worn for these reasons. A quality contact lens fitted by an expert does not produce appalling discomfort and there can be no doubt that eyes with extreme refractive errors see more effectively with such lenses than they do with standard glasses.

The visual field enlarges when unhampered by thick spectacle frames, and the distorting periphery of a thick lens is not used when a lens of equivalent strength is placed upon the eye. Central vision also sharpens, because contact with the eye is a much more natural arrangement than glasses in a frame. The pity is that it is not a more natural corneal arrangement.

Such lenses have their uses for medical reasons. Unilateral aphakics who have normal vision in the other eye may regain binocular function when a contact lens comes near to restoring the optical balance of the eye to what it was before the cataract was removed.

The increasing use of intraocular lens implants has at the moment almost eliminated the optical difficulties of unilateral aphakia.

An abnormal curvature of the cornea (keratoconus) not only induces myopia, but also thin opaque corneal stroma at the summit of the cone. A judiciously designed lens may not only prevent this disaster, but may improve the vision as well and delay the need for corneal grafting. Although it may seem paradoxical there is some evidence that some hard lenses, far from preventing keratoconus, can actually hasten its onset.

When corneal ulcers refuse to heal, stitching the eyelids together (tarsorrhaphy) is not always acceptable, especially in an only eye. A contact lens can be applied as a bandage to allow the corneal epithelium to regenerate without external disturbance.

The lids stay open. The patient may continue to see, and the sceptical will also see that covering the cornea is not just a device to conceal therapeutic defeat.

Contact lens wearers complain from time to time of irritable eyes. This is not surprising as the potential cause has been applied by themselves. Corneal abrasions, erosions, infections and frank assault from trying to remove a contact lens that may not be in position are all ways in which this may happen.

More common is a grumbling conjunctivitis caused by simple intolerance to the lens material, or allergy to the endless variety of solutions available for them to steep in.

Most symptoms will clear away when the lens is taken out. Most symptoms will stay away if the lens is kept out, at least until the signs and any doubts over its suitability have cleared away as well.

Surgical correction

Radial incisions on the deep surface of the cornea were tried by a Japanese eye surgeon, Sato, during the Second World War, to overcome not only a lack of distance vision in their pilots but also a lack of the actual pilots themselves. The kamikaze principle did not make for long careers in the air. At least it spared the pilots the ghastly realization that if they had not given up their lives for the Emperor, they would certainly have given up their eyes.

During the 1970s, Fyodorov, in what was then the Soviet Union, modified this attempt to flatten the corneal curvature by making his attack on the outer surface of the cornea. A computer, fed with appropriate information, instructs the surgeon who then

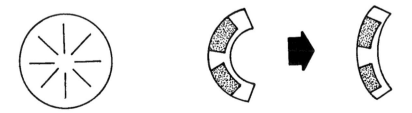

Fig. 2.9   Radial keratotomy – a surgical method of dealing with what might be thought a simple problem. The cornea, weakened by the incisions, bulges and reduces the corneal curvature, thus reducing focusing power.

makes a series of radial incisions around an axial circle as far as the deep corneal layer, and sometimes, alas, beyond.

As can be guessed, the stratagem is not without its drawbacks. Unpleasant reflections can bounce into the eye from the surgical interfaces which act as mirrors. The resultant photophobia might then induce a twinge of regret for the comfortable old glasses, or even the contact lenses. If only it were as effective in severe myopia, it would be accepted without reservation. On the present evidence, it can only be a matter of time before radial keratotomy becomes part of history, like the Mensheviks, an essential catalyst to the start of a revolution, anticipating a new world in which they would play no part.

Photorefractive keratectomy (PRK)

The Excimer laser is the next step in what doubtless will be a sequence of increasing sophistication.

The aim is still to reduce the corneal curvature but without the brutal penetration of its stroma required by radial keratotomy.

With great precision and relative freedom from discomfort, the cornea can be fashioned, within reason, to eliminate spherical or astigmatic refractive errors.

Epikeratophakia

In this technique a living contact lens made of cryolathed corneal material is sutured into the stroma of the cornea. Host epithelium eventually covers the graft, which becomes incorporated into the eye, altering the corneal shape according to its own size. Such a manoeuvre carrying fewer dangers to the developing eye than does a lens implant must have a future in the management of congenital cataract.

Intraocular manipulations

In very high degrees of myopia, surgeons have been moved to counter the strong focusing power of the natural lens with a concave implant into the anterior chamber. An equal surgical interest has been directed at the natural lens itself. Removal of a clear lens, not yet a cataract, reduces the optical myopia enormously but of course does nothing to alter the degenerative areas of myopia which may exist in such eyes.

Both approaches are invasive with all the possible complications of surgical invasion of the eye, made possibly more punitive by flimsy surgical indications to begin with.

SUMMARY

The normally-sighted eye can bring parallel rays of light from the distance to focus on the retina without effort.

The light rays from near objects diverge as they strike the eye and have to be brought to a focus with an effort proportional to the amount of their divergence. The amount of their divergence increases with their proximity. After the mid-forties the hardened lens fails to respond to the ciliary muscles and reading glasses become necessary.

The focal length of the long-sighted eye is too long for the eyeball. Such an eye has to use up its reading focus to see in the distance.

The focal length of the short-sighted eye is too short for the eyeball. Such an eye can never see in the distance at any time, with or without effort.

The astigmatic eye can never properly be in focus either for distance or near because it cannot focus to a point.

The only way for an eye to overcome these errors without glasses is to wrinkle up the eyelids into a slit which, using the principle of a pin-hole camera, puts the eye in focus for anything at any distance.

Unfortunately it also puts the eye in jeopardy for, although a saving may be made at the optician's, a price is paid for this vision that outweighs the cost of a pair of spectacles. It means that no one will ever check for the asymptomatic chronic simple glaucoma.

The physical effort of the eyelids may add interest to the face but will defy all disguising cosmetics.

Yet correcting lenses have never been short of opponents. Even today there are those who fiercely condemn them as an outrage against the body. They offer an ethereal vision to myopes, presbyopes, hypermetropes and astigmatics who are prepared to substitute mystical manoeuvres for spectacles and to return to nature. Any inconvenient hint that the outlines of nature are now perhaps not quite as sharp as they used to be is dismissed as a stumble on the way to eternal truth.

No one would seriously deny that we walk better when we are wearing shoes. If glasses are needed, we will see better when we wear glasses. We do not become addicted to the glasses; we become addicted to the pleasure of seeing.

Yet books are still written to persuade the credulous that an act of will may transform a weakness that they have been born with into a strength they would like. Poor vision has nothing to recommend it at any time, and even less when inflicted needlessly on the gullible with counterfeit promises of visual paradise.

3. What patients complain of and what the complaints signify

Good history taking calls for compassion, diplomacy and editing.

Compassion reminds us that sheer terror is the source of these tortuous descriptions that seem to meander from one insignificant point to the next.

Diplomacy brings with it the gentle skill of cutting short this tangle without giving the slightest hint of impatience.

Editing then allows us to distil what was being confused at length into something clear and brief.

The eye has a very limited response to a multiplicity of insults and patients tend to perceive these responses under five main headings:

1. visual disturbance of some sort
2. double vision
3. pain
4. disturbance of the lacrimal apparatus
5. alteration in appearance.

Only the first two of these are strictly ophthalmic. For the others, normal appearances do not surely need to be read up in a text book and any variations from normal are usually part of daily experience. Pain can occur anywhere. The lacrimal apparatus is really a lubricating gland and drainage system that happens to lie beside the eye.

VISUAL DISTURBANCE

Since the eye is an extension of the brain it makes sense to describe disturbances of vision as we might describe disturbances of the central nervous system:

1. alteration of normal function
2. abnormal features present which should be absent
3. normal features absent which should be present.

ALTERED FUNCTION

Distortion

Imperfection perceived in the centre of vision must raise a question mark over the macula. If no defect is found there, then the next area for suspicion must be the macular fibres of the optic nerve itself. Affection of these are very much the rarity but a Holmesian exclusion of the other possibilities leaves us no other explanation.

Photophobia

Dislike of light is a common indication of unhappy eyes.

The only condition where it pinpoints particular specific pathology is in albinism, where there is insufficient pigment to absorb excess illumination.

Otherwise we find it in patients with generalized viral infections and migraine, who share this dislike of light, and of course neurotics are frequently to be found making public their desire for privacy behind opaque sunglasses.

ABNORMAL FEATURES WHICH SHOULD NOT BE PRESENT

Haloes

Haloes must first of all divide into:

1. those which contain all the colours of the spectrum
2. those which do not.

Spectral haloes are the textbook warning of an eye on or over the brink of acute angle closure.

The mechanism is water retention in the cornea, because a narrow angle obstructs the flow of aqueous. The sodden cornea breaks up white light as does the sky after a rain storm. Because the cornea is round, so is the 'rainbow'.

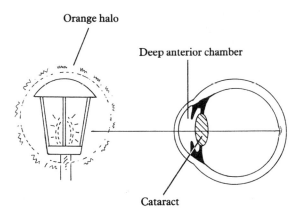

Orange halo

Deep anterior chamber

Cataract

Fig. 3.1 Monochromic haloes mean cataract. A deep anterior chamber means that acute angle closure is impossible.

Haloes of one or two colours are more common than are haloes of all the colours. They mean some sort of opacity and the most likely opacity is cataract.

Haloes are well known from the popular press but that there are two kinds is not so well known. The patient will not make the distinction unless we ask and if we do not ask we will not make the distinction either.

Flashing lights

Visual impulses which focus on the retina in the normal fashion travel along the visual pathway and end up in the occipital cortex as normal vision.

Impulses unfocused on the retina, or indeed any other factor which stimulates the visual fibres, also end up in the visual occipital cortex – not actually as vision, but as a crude version of the same – flashing lights; sometimes phantom images.

Vitreous tugging on the retina is sensed as light flashing, which comes abruptly to an end as the retina is torn.

The lightning streaks of migraine zigzag as part of a well-known sequence.

Stars can appear, float, disappear then reappear when the eyes are turned to the extremes of gaze.

Flashing lights are usually more significant if associated with other symptoms like floaters or actual loss of vision.

Floaters

Because the eye is transparent and the two intraocular cavities full of liquid, opaque particles, by their very movement, justify the term floater. To casual observation all floaters appear the same. They must be identified by their companions.

Simple

The most common, these occur because of degeneration within the vitreous. The hyaluronic acid component, which normally separates invisible vitreal fibres, collapses; the fibres coalesce and become apparent to the patient as little wisps and tendrils – particularly intense against a blue sky or a snowy background, and more so when weariness turns to exhaustion.

Pathological (floaters plus some other feature)

Iritis: Inflammatory flecks dance across the vision at random.
Choroiditis: Choroidal inflammation seeping into the vitreal

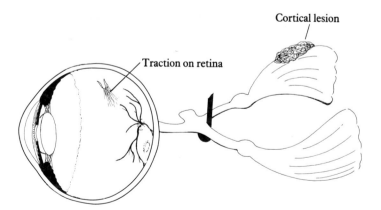

Fig. 3.2   Excitation of the neuro-retina or the visual pathway by any route other than optical will result in a caricature of vision – light flashes if the excitation affects the retina; half-formed phantom figures as the irritation approaches the cerebral cortex.

cavity tends to cause a definite cloud or smudge in the peripheral vision.

Vitreal haemorrhage

Bleeding into the vitreal cavity is generally sudden.

Local causes

1. retinal break
2. retinal break plus detachment
3. diabetic retinopathy
4. hypertensive retinopathy
5. idiopathic haemorrhage

General causes

Must include the bleeding disorders.

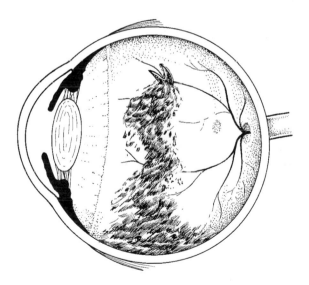

Fig. 3.3   Any opacity in the ocular fluids will move enough to be called a floater. Sudden onset, with added symptoms like flashing lights or visual loss, means that a cause can and must be found. An onset so slow that it is forgotten, with no companion symptoms, means that a cause need not be found and probably will not be.

NORMAL FEATURES WHICH SHOULD BE PRESENT BUT ARE ABSENT

Transient loss of vision (amaurosis fugax)

Defects in the cerebral blood flow or ocular blood flow will produce an instant dimming in the corresponding visual field.

Postural causes where the head rises faster than its blood supply will be obvious from the history.

As for the others, constriction of the great vessels in the neck, possibly exacerbated by hypertension and diabetes, must always be considered.

A raised intraocular pressure can tip the balance against the circulation within the globe when the general circulation is faltering.

Permanent loss of vision

Quiet loss of central vision must make us think of:

1. cataract
2. macular degeneration.

Less common causes lie in:

1. the cornea
2. a retinal detachment creeping up to the macula
3. chronic glaucoma eroding field to the macula
4. optic nerve compression.

Loss of visual field

Any lesion known to general pathology may impinge on the visual pathway. It may not, however, impinge upon consciousness unless it is of sudden onset.

The common sources of field loss in one or both eyes are:

1. chronic glaucoma
2. retinal detachment.

We must not forget the possibility of a homonymous hemianopia almost invariably following a cerebrovascular accident involving the visual pathways. It may occur quietly and be identified in a vague way by the patient as a general decline in vision.

Loss of dark adaptation

Night blindness is not a term that most patients would use but they might admit on questioning that the vision does not adapt to the dark when the lights go out.

If it has followed treatment with widespread photocoagulation for diabetes then the loss might be static. If, however, it is caused by retinal degeneration such as retinitis pigmentosa then in the fullness of time the day vision will go as well, leaving the patient with a tunnel of central vision in a field of darkness.

DOUBLE VISION

Most complaints of double vision turn out to be not double at all but blurred – a distinction that direct questioning will reveal.

Genuine double vision means one of two things:
If it occurs when

1. only one eye is open, then something in the eye – perhaps a cataract – has split the entering light in two.
2. both eyes are open, then some opacity may have still split the light in two but there is also a strong possibility that the eyes have suddenly begun to point in different directions. This also means one of two things:
   a. an extraocular muscle is paralysed
   b. a struggle between the actual ocular balance and the ideal binocular balance has begun to become obvious (latent squint).

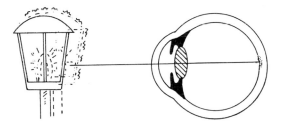

Fig. 3.4   The first question to a patient with double vision is, 'Does it occur with one eye open?' If it does, then the cause is usually an opacity in the transparent structures and the most common opacity is cataract.

Children who squint or adults who started life as children who squinted cannot suffer genuine double vision because they use only one eye at a time.

PAIN

If pain in the eye is caused by the eye then the reason will be obvious in the eye.

Aches in the eye, stabbing pains through the eye, a sensation of pressure behind the eye – such frequent sensations share the common feature that the cause almost invariably lies somewhere else – not infrequently the paranasal sinuses. If pain in the eye is genuinely ocular in origin then there will be:

1. a history of a foreign body
2. a red eye
3. something obvious, like distorted eyelids or eyelashes.

If pain follows the use of the eyes then it is reasonable to ascribe this to some uncorrected refractive error or to some binocular imbalance. Morning headaches are not caused by refractive errors unless insomnia has led to reading all night.

DISTURBANCE OF THE LACRIMAL APPARATUS

People may complain of dry eyes when the lacrimal gland has ceased to produce in later life what it used to produce in early life. The rheumatic disorders are notorious for bringing this about at an earlier age.

Watering may follow excess production or diminished drainage of tears.

Excess production is usually in response to some irritation, like strong wind or infection, and should this be infiltrated with pus, then the water has become a discharge.

Malfunction of the drain can occur for any reason, from ill-fitting eyelids down to obstruction in the nasolacrimal duct. Blockage of the nasolacrimal duct is probably the least common cause of watering.

ALTERATION IN APPEARANCE

Conditions of sudden onset, like a red eye, are beyond doubt. Most people however, fail to recognize gradual changes in their looks. It is left to helpful friends to point out such blemishes. There are several departures from the standard which might be accepted as normal. An inventory of these could be readily constructed and just as readily forgotten. Observation is the thing and, as Sherlock Holmes stated, 'It is not enough to look, we must observe'.

SUMMARY

Loss of vision can be frightening for both the patient and doctor. As the common things are common, reason must not be suspended because the eye is involved, but the important thing in ophthalmology is not always to find out what is wrong but to be sure what is not wrong. To achieve this apparently daunting task all we need to do is to apply the simple unchanging sequence of the seven signs to be described in the next chapter. This system is the basis of the book. To learn it and to practise it bring security to our patients and pleasure to ourselves and also a faint sense of grievance that it should be so simple.

— Double vision usually turns out to be blurred vision.
— Monocular double vision is due to some opacity of the transparent structures.
— Binocular double vision means that some factor either transient or permanent has mechanically taken the eyes beyond the range over which the extraocular muscles normally hold them together.
— *Pain*: If pain in the eye is caused by the eye there will be a sign in the eye.
— *Watering*: A dry eye may become an irritable eye and an irritable eye may water. Simple watering is more often due to a lax eyelid than to blockage of the nasolacrimal duct.
— Cosmetic changes are usually self evident.

To listen to every word our patients utter and to take a complete history is rather like picking every berry before moving on to the next bush – solemnly recommended for other people to do. Of course we must listen and be seen to listen but flabby listening can result in a saga that leaves us no wiser in the end than we were in the beginning.

And of course we must take a history, but 'take' is the vital word. Patients do not know what is important and what is not. It is up to us to tease out the essential strands from their ravelled fear into patterns of essential symptoms. The moment patients are given a free rein to make their own interpretation of symptoms that they have brought to us for our interpretation, then they and we are lost.

4. How to examine the eye

THE SEVEN SIGNS

It is axiomatic in medicine that each body system has its own examination ritual – a check list of observations, rather like that for a broken down car – unchanging and to be followed in order no matter what is thought to be wrong. Indeed that is the whole point of the examination. If we already knew what was wrong, there would be no need for us to look at all unless to find out if something else was wrong as well.

Sadly, the curse of ophthalmology is that it somehow has developed outside medical orthodoxy. Instead of a short check list that never varies, we find a monstrous catalogue of clinical features from which we may select a handful to suit whatever condition we imagine we are going to find. Translate those findings into ophthalmo-babble or dog Latin and it is not to be wondered that ophthalmologists can speak only to each other.

By a strange irony the eye is very easy to examine and it is made easier still by another fact little emphasized. The eye is an organ of limited response to a limitless range of insults. The origin of these responses is described throughout the book and all we need do is learn the same few signs by which we may recognize them.

So, from being an inventory of obscurities, ophthalmic examination reduces to a handful of simple elements:

1. central vision – distance
2. central vision – near
3. field vision
4. cornea
5. pupil
6. anterior chamber depth
7. intraocular pressure.

Then and only then do we come to the ophthalmoscope which sometimes allows a view of the posterior pole of the eye. This could be termed the eighth sign because it should never be considered before the first seven have been checked. In practical terms the posterior pole means the optic disc, the macula and the vessels adjacent to the optic disc.

The direct ophthalmoscope appears easy to learn then turns out to be difficult to use. It has become an emblem – to the ophthalmologist – rather what the stethoscope is to the general practitioner. In common with the stethoscope, it tells us nothing unless we know what we are looking for, and we can only know that by first assembling some signs from the outside.

The 'What do you make of that fundus?' type of examining, particularly favoured in medical wards, leads to stab guessing the universal answer of haemorrhages and exudates, some grade of hypertensive change or, much more likely, to profound and irreversible gloom.

At the root of all ophthalmic teaching lies the assumption that every syndrome is crowned with a unique fundal appearance. That in the presence of aphakia, myopia or cataract it may not be seen with ease, that it may not be seen at all and that it is certainly not unique are somehow never mentioned.

In time the fundal appearance becomes a shorthand for the whole clinical picture and the fundus remains as invisible and uninformative as ever.

The answer is to accept that we will see nothing with the ophthalmoscope until we know what we are looking for. When we get to the point of knowing what we should see, then after a while we may even begin to see it. The role of the ophthalmoscope, like the role of the stethoscope, is to confirm what we expect to find. It is not a diagnostic flourish all on its own.

TESTS FOR CENTRAL VISION

Distance

Most medical establishments can produce a Snellen chart of sorts – usually a yellow heirloom where the letters fade into the background and which at 6 metres could be mistaken for a Cubist painting. The ideal demands sharp black letters on a clear white background in good illumination.

The letters on the chart reduce in size, step by step, from those which ought to be seen at 60 metres to those which ought to be seen at 4 metres by the normal eye.

The gradation is worked out on the principle that to the eye a letter from the 6 metre line seen at 6 metres, will appear to have the same size as a letter from the 12 metre line seen at 12 metres.

Since the test is conducted at 6 metres, then standard vision recorded as 6/6 (20/20 ft) means that the eye at 6 metres sees a letter that ought to be seen at 6 metres.

Failure to make out the letters at the correct distance does not necessarily mean that the eyes are defective. They may simply need a pair of spectacles. The question is – how do we prove it?

The pinhole disc

The answer is a pinhole – an ingenious device – the principles of which were first described by a Jesuit priest in the early seventeenth century but which were probably known much earlier. Visual loss due to refractive error corrects with the pinhole. Visual loss due to something else does not.

In any optical system, peripheral rays are bent towards a focusing point by that system, but there is always a central ray that passes through undeviated, because there is nothing to deviate it.

In the normal-sighted eye this central ray doesn't matter greatly, because all other rays will reach a point focus at the macula. On the other hand, in eyes with gross refractive error, peripheral rays

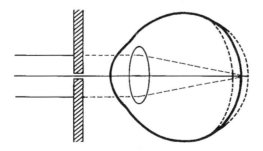

Fig. 4.1   Every bundle of rays from every point is reduced to one ray and each one of them is in focus. The ray through the macula is the vital clinical one. If the central vision improves with a pinhole, it can improve with glasses.

will not come near the macula and they overwhelm the central one that does.

The pinhole disc eliminates all these rays and allows the central one to pass on its own. If the macula has the potential to see, then the pinhole disc will prove it.

Of course bundles of light reduced to one undeviated ray pass through the pinhole from all points in the visual field, but the macular ray is the one we are after.

The pinhole disc may have one drawback. The hole has to be small. It may be hard for the elderly to find and once they have found it they may then proceed to lose it.

A disc of multiple pinholes gets round these problems. Many holes are easier to find than is one hole and a wavering hand will manage to place one of them on the axial line.

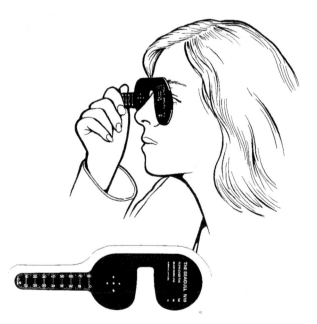

Fig. 4.2 The disc with the pinhole should be held about one inch (2.5 cm) before the eye. Leaning on the cheek keeps it steady. Multiple pinholes do not place such a premium on steadiness. And usually one will be found by the patient. The pinhole can be used for near vision as well. The capacity to make out the smallest print, despite a poor performance for distance, indicates an intact macula. No improvement with a pinhole means the problem is not a refractive error.

Each eye has to be examined separately, with the patient holding the disc just clear of the eyelashes.

Near vision

This test of course demands an element of focus from the normal-sighted eye, and a greater element of focus from the long-sighted eye. The short-sighted eye requires no effort because it is focused for near anyway.

The long-sighted eye may have used up all its reading focus in the distance; the presbyopic eye has no focusing range to use up.

The pinhole comes to our rescue again, as it bypasses all refractive errors.

Near vision is not just a proximal version of distance vision. The eye for all sorts of reasons may not make out the Snellen chart with ease, if at all. However, if it can make out small print, then we can assume that the macula is working to some degree. Yet how often are patients dismissed as 'blind', and their eyes useless, because someone has measured the distance vision only and found it to be not very good.

To avoid confusing patients and occasionally ourselves, it is best to use the term 'reading' for near and 'seeing' for distance. There is an understandable tendency to ask people what they can read on the Snellen chart and then watch them struggle with their reading glasses before we pick up what they are trying to do.

VISION NOT RECORDABLE

Failure to discriminate the biggest Snellen letter or the largest reading print does not necessarily mean that the eye is lost. Vision is then graded:

1. counting fingers – CF
2. hand movements – HM
3. perception of light – PL.

Light perception with clear media is generally beyond improvement.

However, light perception with a dense cataract can often be turned into excellent vision by simple extraction. Just how excellent will depend obviously on the state of the retina. If the eye is aware of light in the four quadrants of the visual field then all things being equal it has nothing to lose by cataract extraction.

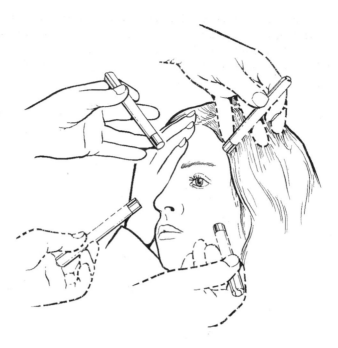

Fig. 4.3   A dense cataract might stop the peripheral retina from picking up hand movements in the visual field. It would need to be exceedingly dense to prevent awareness of light in the four quadrants.

TESTS FOR FIELD VISION

Erosion of the peripheral field can often continue unchecked because most people are not aware that there is any vision other than central. Even if they were aware they would baulk at the concept of two monocular cones of vision, overlapping in a binocular circle.

The visual pathways

These run anatomically from the retinae along the optic nerves, the optic chiasma, the optic tracts and the optic radiations to the occipital cortex of the brain.

Each visual field is split into a temporal half and a nasal half. This split takes place vertically through a fixing point of central vision. The temporal half of each retina is represented in the visual cortex of its own side. The nasal part of each retina crosses over to the opposite side at a junction known as the optic chiasma. It then continues backwards to be represented in the occipital cortex opposite. The chiasma is very closely related to the pituitary gland and the internal carotid artery.

The arrangement is simpler than it looks and it clearly has a purpose beyond that of tormenting those who try to understand it. Everything picked up by the retina is seen in the opposite field. Thus objects on the floor will be seen by the upper retina, those on the roof by the lower retina, and so on around the field.

The visual field on the right side does not depend on the right eye alone. The temporal half of that field is served by:

1. the right nasal retina
2. the left temporal retina.

This image is a vital one because patients frequently describe visual loss on the right side as being visual loss in the right eye. The fact that the left eye could also be involved is somehow too baffling to contemplate.

It must now be obvious that the visual pathways split quite distinctively into three sections:

1. The optic nerve from the chiasma forwards serves the one eye carrying the fibres for:
    a. the large temporal field (nasal retina)
    b. the smaller nasal field (temporal retina)
    c. macular function.
2. At the chiasma, the nasal fibres from the nasal retinae (temporal fields) cross. They lie at the posterior fork of the chiasma beside the macular fibres. Pressure in this area can cause:
    a. bitemporal field loss
    b. bilateral macular loss.
    It is at the chiasma that lesions, usually compressive, can give rise to mirror image defects on opposite sides of the body.
3. The fibres behind the chiasma pass the lateral geniculate body and sweep as optic radiations into the occipital cortex. Lesions along this line – either compressive or ischaemic – affect the temporal fibres from one eye plus the nasal fibres from the other eye. They will therefore produce a field defect on one side of the body which will be detectable in both the left eye and the right eye (homonymous).

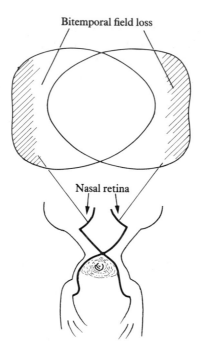

Fig. 4.4   The temporal field is supplied by the nasal retina. The fibres which cross in the chiasma are vulnerable to pressure from an enlarged pituitary gland. It is at the chiasma that one lesion can affect both sides of the body. The hand movement field test, carried out as described, will pick up such temporal loss. However, flapping the hands halfway between the patient and the doctor will not.

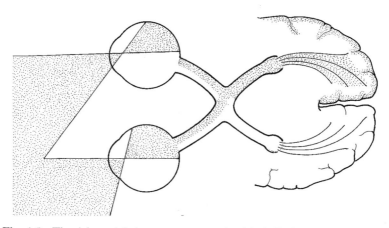

Fig. 4.5   The right occipital cortex represents the right half of each retina and the left half of the visual field. The fibres from the nasal retina of each eye have to cross at the chiasma. A lesion behind the chiasma produces a field defect on the opposite side of the body – a homonymous hemianopia – one lesion, one side (opposite).

The visual field takes on the shape of a cone of buckshot discharged from an asymmetrical blunderbuss flaring forwards and sideways, upwards and downwards.

The diameter of each monocular cone widens to infinity as it sprays from the eye, achieving infinite width on the horizon where of course it is too wide to allow any sensible assessment.

To make a consistent estimate of its border we have to pick it up at the same point each time, rather nearer than at infinity:

— 5 cm from the lateral orbital margin
— 5 cm in front of the fellow eye
— 5 cm from the chin
— 5 cm from the junction of the forehead with the scalp.

Each normal monocular cone has:

1. an outer contour – the peripheral limits of vision
2. an inner quality – a sensitivity dependent on the:
   a. size, colour and brightness of objects visualized
   b. surrounding illumination.

Any areas of blunted sensitivity can be thought of as empty spaces, free of buckshot, within the cone.

TESTING THE OUTER CONTOUR

The hand movement field (confrontation)

As with microscopy we start with low magnification for an overall impression and in most circumstances this is all we need.

The aim of this hand movement test is to pick up the peripheral edges of the visual cone of each eye separately.

The patient is asked to cover one eye with the flat of the hand and to fix on the examiner's eye or nose or whatever seems more riveting.

It makes matters easier for patients if we first show them what we are looking for – a shimmering movement of the fingers on a fixed hand and wrist.

We then take this movement gently from the seeing inside of the cone to the non-seeing outside and back again, identifying the dividing line on the way.

There are other ways of attempting to elicit this information and they all share two features – they are complicated and uninformative. Traditional theory demands that we compare our field with that of the patient. Such an approach makes two dangerous assumptions:

— How do we know that the fields are comparable?
— How do we know that our fields are normal?

If these weaknesses are not enough there is an even bigger defect. If the patient is set some 2–3 feet away from us, our hand wagging halfway between on the temporal side misses the vital outer 30° of the visual field. It means that the examiner and the patient could both be harbouring pituitary tumours nibbling away at their temporal fields, and each be blissfully unaware that anything was wrong.

When patients complain of sore feet we do not remove our own shoes, but the classic confrontation test seems to be based on this principle. In practice it imposes so many difficulties on us that we have no conscious mind left to interpret what we see.

We forget that the patient's head can swivel upwards, so we come down to their eye level in a half crouch. Our attempts to cover one eye leave us with one hand short. We take refuge in winking which, coupled with the missing hand and the half flexed

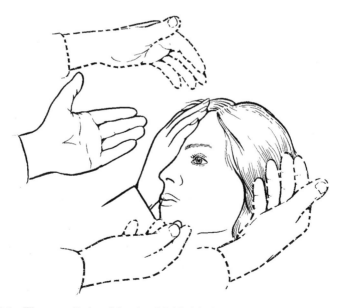

Fig. 4.6   The outer limits of the visual field picked up with hand movements.

knees, might give the impression that the test had been devised to make us appear ridiculous and the field of defect not appear at all. The only indication of normal vision on the part of the patient is then the barely suppressed laughter.

THE INNER QUALITY

The perception of the visual field within the limits of its margins is something that can vary from person to person and indeed from disease to disease. A study of this is best left to those with a special interest in the eye, but one or two features mentioned now might well make them at least familiar when they are mentioned later in the book.

Although the shimmering fingers can be picked up at the outer limits of the cone, something smaller might be missed within these limits.

Such a defect within the visual field has been called a scotoma too long for the name to be dropped. They can be detected by a variety of methods, all resembling each other more than they differ.

The essence is to present to the eye a target large enough to be picked up by the normal field but small enough not to be seen by the unhealthy field.

Such variation in intensity can be achieved by altering the

— *size*
— *colour*
— *illumination*

of the object – and the

— *background* against which the defects are looked for.

We can sometimes find, within the field of vision, areas that will lose a small target but find a larger one. We call these 'relative defects'.

The concept is perhaps best understood if we imagine someone in the jungle visually fixing on something motionless – a snake for example. If there were a defect in the temporal field of vision, it might be extensive enough to allow a monkey to frolic unseen but not a gorilla. As dusk settled even the gorilla might disappear. Such a defect would be 'relative'.

Were the gorilla invisible in all illuminations then the defect would be 'absolute'.

TESTING THE INNER QUALITY

Moving targets (kinetic perimetry)

Pins with red and white heads are frequently to be found in medical wards, plucked from lapels to plot defects inside the field of vision. In skilled hands they can yield much information although they take no account of variations in the background or in the state of illumination. Less skilled hands are much more likely to be perforated by the sharp end.

Bjerrum screen

White targets are moved against a uniform black background in uniform illumination. Like so much else in ophthalmology it helps if we know what we are looking for and there is a tendency nowadays to use more expensive devices.

The supreme advantages of the Bjerrum screen are simplicity and an absence of moving parts that might break down.

The Mutlukan–Cullen Test

When conduction in the visual pathways from the disc backwards falters, the field supplied by the affected fibres does not perceive

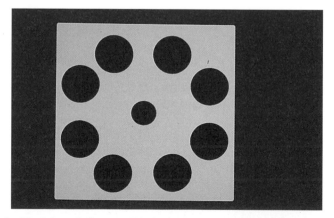

Fig. 4.7   Mutlukan–Cullen test. Diminished perception of red follows conduction defects in the optic nerve which themselves sometimes follow compression or demyelination.

the colour 'red' as the brilliant hue perceived in the normal field. Sometimes it does not perceive it at all.

Until now, such discrepancies in red perception have been searched for with red headed pins or with the Bjerrum screen. Unfortunately, those very patients about whose visual pathways we require to be so informed are the very ones who cannot or will not be bothered with pins or screens.

The principle of the test is based on a series of red dots circling round a fixation point. When the card with the dots is held at the reading distance and the eye fixed on the central point, the circle of dots stimulates the retina wide of the macula.

In homonymous hemianopia there is total absence of perception in the affected field. Compressive lesions of the optic nerve may leave the contours intact but the quality within reduced – a reduction in sensitivity proportional to reduction in red perception.

This test incorporates all that is informative about the principle of comparisons, without the incitement to mutiny. A card held at the normal reading position could well seem less threatening to patients whose perceptive defects might lead them to see menace when we are only trying to demonstrate if they see at all.

Although in the presence of colour blindness its findings would be open to question, its inexpensive simplicity, which ought to lead to its universal adoption, will doubtless do the opposite.

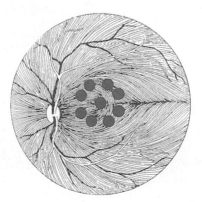

Fig. 4.8   Mutlukan–Cullen test – the area of retina stimulated.

The Goldman perimeter

This machine explores the entire extent of the visual field. The head is placed inside a cup – a third of a metre across and shaped like the retina brandy goblet, but pointing in the other direction. It offers uniformity and accuracy but with a moving target. It induces a sense of unreality, with one's head appearing to be entering a space machine.

Moving eye

Damato field test

Of recent invention, this ingenious contrivance utilizes what patients want to do most – use their central fixation and move their eyes. All other tests demand that the cups remain still.

With the other eye covered they are asked to follow the numbers from 1–26; this has the effect of running the central black dot over their visual field within the margins of the cone. If the black dot is visible at all times, there is no scotoma.

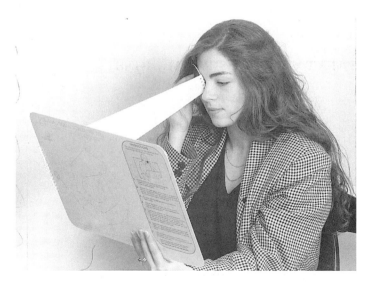

Fig. 4.9   The Damato field test.

The field analysers

Static perimetry

Here the targets do not move but rather flash on and off. There can certainly be little ambiguity about whether the targets are seen or not. The danger here is that these tests can be made so sensitive that they may uncover defects that may not actually exist but which once mentioned can induce irreversible anxiety and can be the starting point for a galaxy of pointless neurological investigations and for frequent requests for an ophthalmic opinion.

The essential part of the visual field examination is to determine the margins of the visual cone. If a defect is discovered then a host of experts will rush in to investigate the inner quality.

If defects (scotomata) exist within a normal visual cone, then other signs should prevent us from missing them.

INATTENTION

Patients with lesions of the parietal lobe may have deficiency in perception without actual loss of perception. When both the temporal and nasal field are tested at the same time, that field which corresponds to the damaged parietal lobe will give the impression of extinction. If each quadrant is tested separately then the danger of recording a defect that does not exist will be eliminated.

THE NEXT THREE ESSENTIAL SIGNS

These must be observed every time. Continued repetition will in a little while make this examination ritual second nature. There are not after all many elements to remember. One leads on to the next and indeed after a while all three may be made at once. They are:

1.   the state of the cornea
2.   the state of the pupil
3.   the depth of the anterior chamber.

THE STATE OF THE CORNEA

The front surface of the cornea glistens and sparkles in youth, turning in time into the familiar lack-lustre eyes of the elderly – as though decades of watching human activity have dulled the eye as well as the spirits.

A white circle (the arcus senilis) separated from the sclera by a small gap of clear cornea, may give the impression of reduction in ocular size. Except in those rare patients with raised triglycerides,

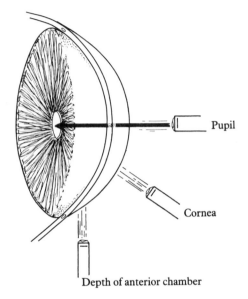

Depth of anterior chamber

Fig. 4.10   The cornea, the pupil and the anterior chamber – the second group of three signs. Coupled with the finger tension, they form a brisk and efficient way of distinguishing the three serious red eyes from each other and from all the rest.

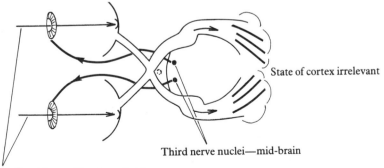

Fig. 4.11   The pupil reflexes. Light presented to one eye constricts both pupils. One of the common causes of a sluggish pupil reflex is a dying battery.

it does not give any worthwhile information about the general state of serum lipids.

Breaches in the corneal epithelium, either by an abrasion or by infection, will be apparent in the light of a torch as a certain roughness. The area of roughness can be accurately delineated with a dye known as sodium fluorescein, which stains very precisely the cornea where the epithelium is missing. A small magnifying lens makes these observations easier and may give them a certain professional air.

Sodium fluorescein

Coming as either a liquid or as an impregnated strip of paper, this is another easily carried piece of equipment. The liquid perhaps is less happy in use than the strip, because as well as staining the eye it will stain everything else it touches.

In theory the paper should be moistened with some sterile isotonic solution, but water from the tap is quite acceptable. A red eye may be so moist anyway that extra wetting may be needless. The tip can then be stroked along the inner surface of the lower lid, allowing the dye to fill the conjunctival sac.

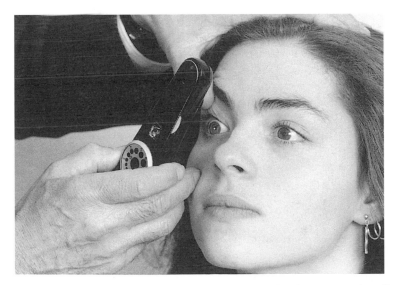

Fig. 4.12 Using the ophthalmoscope as a torch to examine the cornea and pupil.

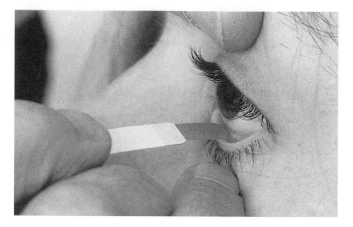

Fig. 4.13   Using a fluorescein dye strip.

A green coloration will now wash across the cornea, picking up in special detail any areas where the corneal epithelium is gone.

THE STATE OF THE PUPIL

The pupil is that hole in the centre of the iris which changes in size in response to stimuli. It has two muscles. The more powerful, a sphincter running around its margin, makes the pupil smaller when it contracts and larger when it relaxes. Active constriction is mediated via the parasympathetic nervous system.

The weaker muscle – the dilator – runs from this round muscle outwards towards the root of the iris. Active dilatation, mediated via the sympathetic nervous system, reinforces the dilatation started by the relaxing sphincter.

The pupil regulates the amount of light entering the eye, constricting in sunlight, dilating at dusk and decreasing in size when active near vision is called for to allow a greater precision of focus.

Thus there are two distinct reflex pathways:

1.   the response to light
2.   the response to near focus (accommodation).

The former is by far the more important.

The light reflex

As with other reflexes we have a neuromuscular response to a stimulus, an inflow pathway and an outflow pathway.

The stimulus is light which, falling on the retina, triggers impulses which travel by the optic nerve along the optic tract to the lateral geniculate body at the level of the mid-brain. Because the inflow does not rise above this level the pupil reflexes can remain intact, although destruction of the occipital cortex has made the patient blind.

The inflow begins with the retina and optic nerve, then splits at the chiasma, whence its impulses pass on to the third nerve nucleus of each side.

The outflow begins with the third nerve nucleus, passing along the third nerve to the ciliary ganglion and finally to the pupil.

Because half the fibres from each eye cross at the chiasma, bright light falling on one eye will constrict the pupils of both.

The test

The pupil, confronted with the bright light constricts briskly and remains constricted. If there is any defect in perception in the retina or conduction along the optic nerve, the second half of this reflex alters and the pupil keeps breaking open again.

This 'relative afferent pupillary defect', contracted to RAPD, is not uncommon during or following an attack of optic neuritis. The commonest cause of a diminished light reflex is probably failing conduction within the torch battery rather than in the optic nerve.

Inflow defect

Dysfunction at any point on the inflow pathway diminishes or eliminates the inflow stimulus on that side. The result is a diminished or absent constriction of the pupil on the affected side (direct reflex) and on the opposite side (consensual reflex).

Outflow defect

Dysfunction at any point on the outflow pathway will result in diminished or absent constriction on the affected side, no matter which eye is illuminated.

The swinging light test

When the light is directed at one pupil, both pupils constrict – all things being equal. The first constriction is called the direct light reflex; the second pupil constriction is called the consensual reflex.

However, to observe the consensual reflex, we have to illuminate that pupil also, thereby adding a direct component to any consensual elements that we might observe.

Swinging the light from one pupil to the next in a wide circle rather than in a direct line allows us to observe the consensual constriction giving way before direct constriction takes over.

State of cortex irrelevant

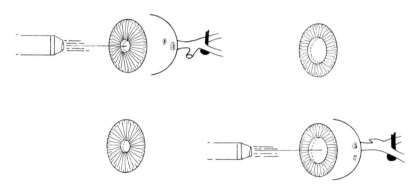

Fig. 4.14   In-flow defect. Light presented to the healthy eye (**left**) constricts both pupils. Light presented to the affected eye (**right**) constricts neither.

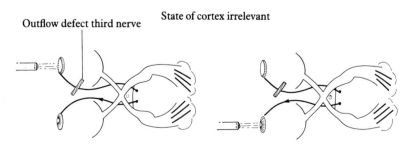

Outflow defect third nerve   State of cortex irrelevant

Fig. 4.15   Outflow defect. Light presented to the affected eye (**left**) constricts only the pupil on the normal side. Light presented to the normal eye (**right**) still constricts the same pupil.

The accommodation reflex

Although clearly there must be an inflow pathway, it is as yet unknown despite much imaginative speculation. It has been suggested that contraction of the medial rectus muscles, when the eyes converge to read, sparks off the inflow impulse. The outflow must be considered the same as that of the light reflex.

THE DEPTH OF THE ANTERIOR CHAMBER

The eclipse test

The anterior chamber is that space between the iris and the cornea. If it is deep, the iris is gently convex – almost a plane. If it is shallow, the iris is grossly convex – almost like a hillock with the pupil at its summit and one slope hidden from the other, or perhaps like the back of a hand, first extended then flexed.

This concealment, progressive as the anterior chamber becomes more shallow, is the basis of the eclipse test.

The test is critical:

1. to tell us when it is safe to dilate the pupil
2. to detect people, as yet symptomless, who might be in danger from acute angle closure.

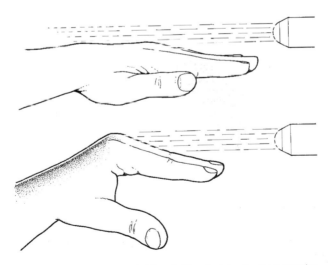

Fig. 4.16 The back of an extended hand, like the iris of a deep anterior chamber, can be illuminated. That of a flexed hand, like the iris of a shallow chamber, cannot.

A light aimed from the margin of the cornea across the iris plane will illuminate as much of the anterior chamber as its depth allows. In a deep anterior chamber the entire iris will be suffused with light.

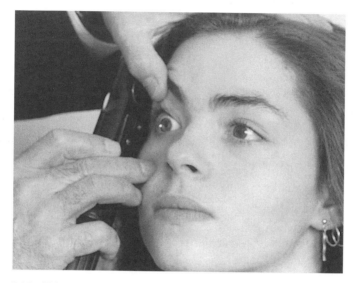

Fig. 4.17   Using the ophthalmoscope as a torch to determine the depth of the anterior chamber – the eclipse test.

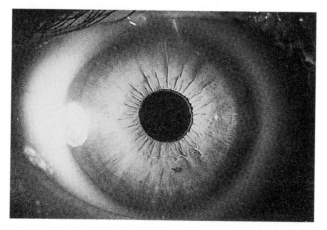

Fig. 4.18   Eclipse test negative – the anterior chamber is deep and none of the iris in shadow. The pupil may be dilated with impunity.

In a shallow anterior chamber – the kind that may give lead to acute angle closure – only the half adjacent to the light will be illuminated: the remote half is in shadow. The light is eclipsed.

THE SEVENTH SIGN

INTRAOCULAR PRESSURE

Thoughts of acute angle closure should bring to mind an eye in which more aqueous has been secreted than has been excreted. However, to think that the intraocular pressure is raised is not enough. We have to prove it.

Tonometry is the name given to this manoeuvre, whether it be done by the fingers or by instruments. The latter are best left to those who are prepared to spend much time mastering them. The former is more accurate if a little time is spent mastering it as well.

Digital tonometry

We palpate the eye as we would a boil. Clearly it cannot be done on the globe directly and the manoeuvre has to be carried out through the eyelid. The critical thing is to palpate the eye and not the tarsal plate. Palpation therefore must be done above the tarsal

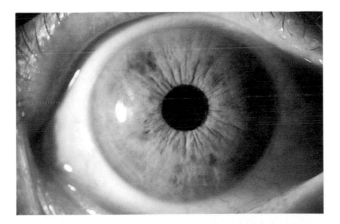

Fig. 4.19 Eclipse test positive – the iris surface remote from the beam is in shadow. Angle closure possible. Pupil not to be dilated by topical or systemic medications.

plate with the eye looking downwards. The eyelid is at its thinnest just under the upper outer angle of the orbit.

The easiest way is to lean on the patient's forehead with the sides of the ring and little fingers. This stabilizes the hand and releases the middle or index fingers for palpation.

The palpating fingers brush together pulp to nail. They must maintain contact with each other and with the globe. One finger is active. One is passive. One finger is mobile and the other static. The mobile finger presses gently on the eye with a tiny alternating action whilst the static finger senses the thrill of fluctuation. The softer the eye the greater the fluctuation.

To press with both fingers would tell us nothing. To lift one off altogether would tell us less.

In the days when a knowledge of Latin indicated a well-spent youth, the shortcomings of the test were glossed over with the classical tag 'Tactus eruditis'.

Rough though it may seem, it is more precise than tonometry done badly with an instrument, and fingers are not in need of regular calibration.

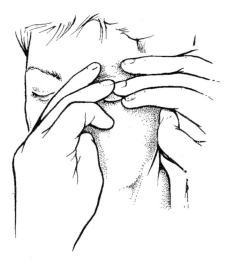

Fig. 4.20   Not everyone has access to a tonometer. The hands lean on the forehead, while the index or middle fingers are held firmly together pulp to nail and firmly on the eye above the lateral end of the tarsal plate. A slight movement of one finger sets up a shimmer of fluctuation that is sensed by the other finger. This technique may record 'hard' by mistake but never 'soft' by mistake.

Clearly a little practice will make us familiar with the feel of the normal eye, but a lot more practice is required to achieve comparable accuracy with an instrument.

If a tonometer is wrong, it could read either high or low, and it is not more scientific just because an error is recorded in millimetres of mercury.

If the fingers get it wrong, they are almost certain to err on the high side. Such a mistake may lead to needless referrals; it will not lead to blindness.

THE EIGHTH SIGN

OPHTHALMOSCOPY: LOOKING AT THE FUNDUS

We come at last to the direct ophthalmoscope. Ophthalmoscopy became fashionable just before the American Civil War when Helmholtz rediscovered in Berlin what had first been described in Breslau 30 years previously by Purkinje – a man whose entire life seems to have been spent making discoveries that brought distinction to others.

The idea was brilliant and it led ophthalmology out of the dark ages in more ways than one. Light is passed in through the pupil, reflected by the red choroid and picked up on its way out through a small peep-hole which blocks the passage of all other reflected light. Were everyone normal sighted it would be as simple as that,

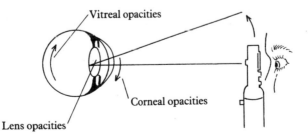

Fig. 4.21 Opacities are best seen through the dilated pupil against the red reflex. When the observer and his ophthalmoscope move slightly from side to side, any opacities will move by parallax. Those in the cornea will move against the light. Those in the vitreous will move with the light. Those in the lens will not move at all.

and simpler still through a dilated pupil. However, refractive errors in both doctor and patient make it less simple again.

Each ophthalmoscope must contain a disc of lenses which can be rotated clockwise to compensate for long sight, or anticlockwise to compensate for short sight. Clockwise rotation pulls the focus up towards the instrument. Anticlockwise rotation pushes the focus back to the retina.

The bespectacled ophthalmoscopist can chose to wear or not to wear glasses. If they are discarded their strength has to be rotated into the ophthalmoscope – clockwise for long sight, anticlockwise for short sight.

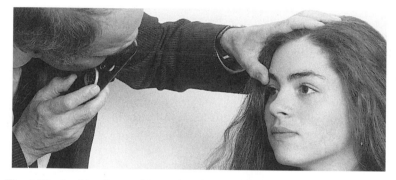

Fig. 4.22   Looking for opacities against the red reflex.

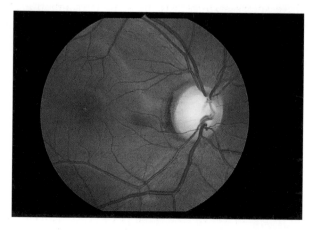

Fig. 4.23   Normal fundus – African with choroidal markings obscured by pigment retina. The disc shows physiological cupping that might be graded 0.3.

The direct ophthalmoscope is versatile. It can be used as a light source, and it can also be used to detect opacities in the cornea, the lens and the vitreous. It is by far the best way to demonstrate cataract.

With the instrument set at two notches clockwise, light is directed at the patient's eye from a distance of 20 cm (8 in). The pupil, especially when dilated, will fill with the red reflex from the choroid. Any opacities will then show up against this red glow and their position can be determined by simple parallax.

When the ophthalmoscope is moved slightly from side to side certain opacities will appear to move as well, but in different directions.

Opacities in:

1. the cornea will move against the light
2. the lens will not move at all
3. the vitreous will move with the light.

The inside of the eye baffles many people because they are uncertain how to look at it, and equally uncertain what to look at. They almost expect a diagnosis to appear just because they have managed to get the retina in focus, and in myopes and aphakics it is not always easy even to do that.

The classic background appearance of the fundus is the product of four layers vying for the attention of the ophthalmoscopist. The appearance is quite different when a pathologist has cut the eye in half.

The white sclera struggles to be seen through the choroid, which overlays it with red. The pigment retina will then darken this red/white amalgam sometimes regularly, sometimes not, and the amount of darkening will depend on the amount of pigment.

The fundus of an albinoid myope will be almost white, whilst that of a Somali hypermetrope will be almost mallard-duck green. In both, the neuro-retina is transparent when flat face on but grey when detached and seen in profile.

Pupil not dilated

It is not always convenient to wait for a mydriatic to paralyse the pupil sphincter, and we are frequently called upon to shine a bright light into the eye whilst a brisk pupil reflex is trying to keep it out. An ophthalmic opinion through the undilated pupil is worthless but since it is attempted so frequently we might as well mention en passant that the only thing liable to be seen is the optic nerve head, and not always that.

As the optic nerves angle into the eye from the chiasma, we have a better chance of picking them up by directing the beam 'towards the pituitary gland'. The tempting straight on position floods the macula with light, constricts the pupil and leaves us wondering how anyone can ever see anything at the back of the eye and how we might hide our discomfiture from the patient.

Patients do not help either, because they feel that following the light and the examiner somehow assists in the examination, a mistake discovered just before both end up on the floor. Opacities in the media, particularly at an age when the pupil becomes smaller still, heighten discomfiture into paralytic despair.

Pupil dilated

Should the history suggest that a fundal view is obligatory, then the pupil must be dilated with some short-acting drug that paralyses the parasympathetic system. Tropicamide wears off in 2–3 hours. Cyclopentolate lasts somewhat longer. An old bottle of homatropine is to be found in most ward cupboards and should be thrown out before it has a chance to paralyse a patient's focus for some days – an intolerable burden, especially if dilatation of the pupil has failed to produce a diagnosis to boot.

As well as homatropine lurking in the ward cupboard, there lurks in everyone's subconscious the notion that dilating drops

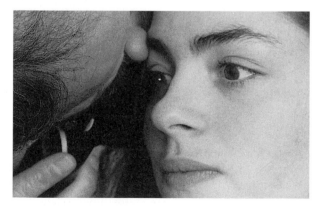

Fig. 4.24   Examining the fundus.

should never be used if the patient has 'glaucoma'. This translates into practice that they should never be used at all – an embargo strengthened by data sheets which so often include 'glaucoma' in their contraindications. These data sheets are compiled by people who do not know that 'glaucoma' has at least six meanings.

The embargo applies only to eyes with a possible tendency to acute angle closure – eyes with a shallow anterior chamber, where dilatation of the pupil may suddenly block the angle. Should the eclipse test indicate a deep anterior chamber, as it usually will, then the pupil may be dilated and it need not be constricted afterwards.

The next temptation to be resisted is to gaze at the entire fundus at once. The direct ophthalmoscope, even in the most practised hands, can rarely reach beyond the equator of the eye. In fact the equator may be defined as the limits of view of the direct ophthalmoscope through the dilated pupil. It is therefore at its best around the posterior pole, where three main features come into view:

1. the optic disc (the papilla or optic nerve head)
2. the macula
3. the retinal vessels.

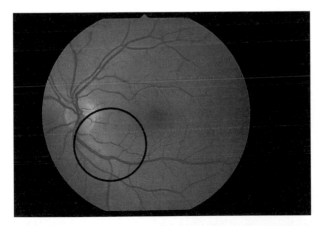

Fig. 4.25 Normal fundus. What is normal varies from race to race. The features to look for are: the disc (margin, colour, cup); the macula, which should be regular, dark and round on the temporal side of the optic nerve head; the blood vessels, which should show no variation in arterial calibre or nipping at the arteriovenous crossings. The fundal landscape is seen with the direct ophthalmoscope in small, circular segments.

The optic disc

Although measuring some 1.5 mm across, the optic disc appears three times that when looked at with the ophthalmoscope. It appears larger still in large myopic eyes and smaller in hypermetropic eyes.

It presents three main features which devotees of cricket might remember with the letters MCC. For those who regard cricket as the Englishman's substitute for philosophy, such metaphysical associations might make the letters more memorable.

M — The *margin* should be sharp in normal eyes, but in small crowded eyes might well be blurred.

C — The *colour* will vary according to the size of the eye. It will be pale in the myope where the optic nerve head capillaries are more spaciously distributed. In the hypermetrope it will appear a darker red for the opposite reason.

C — The *cup*, or *cavity*, in the centre of the disc takes up about a quarter of its size. As a concession to metrication, descriptions have now become decimal and the fashionable term is now cup–disc ratio. If no cup is apparent, the ratio is 0:0. If virtually nothing but cup is apparent, the ratio is 0:8 or more.

The macula

The absolute centre of this highly sensitive retina – the fovea – lies some 1.5 disc diameters temporal to the optic nerve head. It lies in a pit where the retinal layers shelve to allow the maximal amount of light to fall upon the foveal cones and it is seen as a glistening dot in the young eye. The area around the dot is heaped up and somewhat thicker than the peripheral retina. Though red, it is a rather darker red than that of its surroundings.

Because all the features seem to be variations on the red theme, it can be helpful sometimes if red can be eliminated. The green filter of the ophthalmoscope is given the name 'red-free' because it eliminates the red choroidal glow that dominates the fundal view.

Blood vessels become black, the disc a ghostly silver-green and the ocular layers seem to stand apart from each other. The normal macula appears as a dark, round smudge. The abnormal macula appears as anything but a regular dark, round smudge.

In ordinary white light, the normal and the abnormal might look the same.

The retinal vessels

The central retinal artery emerges from the optic disc to spread as arterioles branching and tapering over the entire fundus. Its capillaries feed that half of the neuro-retina adjacent to the vitreous, and blood is returned by the retinal venules which follow the line of the arterioles back into the optic disc. The central retinal artery is an end-vessel anastomosing with no other arterial system.

The arterioles and venules can be seen forming an arcade around the macula. The words 'arteries' and 'veins' and their diminutives tend to be interchanged rather casually.

SUMMARY

There are only seven essential signs – two groups of three, plus one. They lead from one to the other in a sequence, which reasonably begins with vision and gathers in its own momentum.

1. *Central vision* – for *distance*
2. *Central vision* – for *near*
   The pinhole disc substitutes for glasses. The ability to read the smallest print confirms a functioning macula, even though performance with the distance chart is not impressive.
3. *Field vision* – its extent 5 cm from the body every time brings a sense of uniformity to what we find. The test is not crude, but it may sometimes be done crudely.
4. *Cornea* – the epithelium should glisten and sparkle evenly and sodium fluorescein can mark out the areas where it does not.
5. *Pupil* – the light reflex may be demonstrated with the same torch used to examine the cornea.
6. *Anterior chamber* – with the cornea on one side and the pupil on the other, it requires no great feat of memory to remember that the anterior chamber is in between.
7. *Finger tension* – if the anterior chamber brings the intraocular pressure to mind, it should next bring the globe itself to the fingers.

The ocular movements need not be looked at unless the history suggests some defect in the extraocular muscles. Such an examination is not actually ophthalmic but belongs by right to the cranial nerves.

Only at this point should we think of looking at the retina with the ophthalmoscope, and even that should be delayed until any

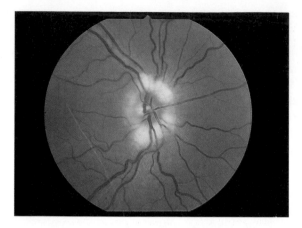

Fig. 4.26   Myelinated nerve fibres – an integral part of retinal development which has usually vanished by birth. Occasionally, fragments remain behind.

opacities in the cornea, lens or vitreous have been established. The whole point of the fundal examination is to recognize within the eye what our findings outside the eye have led us to expect.

To be resisted is the notion that all ophthalmic problems will yield at once to the ophthalmoscope without any prior examination. It is an idea fostered in medical wards, where residents, struggling against the pupil, the sunlight and total ignorance of the eye's performance, would be publicly derided as models of incompetence were they so to use their stethoscope out of order.

An eye at risk

The eye is an organ of limited responses.

The secret of sleeping easily on lonely decisions is to recognize that although many influences can damage the eye, each part of the eye tends to respond in the same way every time. As long as we can recognize that something has happened we work out the cause later.

An equally important finding often in the face of anxiety, apparent disaster and threats of more to come is that, in fact, nothing serious has happened.

While it is ideal to know what is wrong it is often practically extremely helpful to know what is not wrong.

As long as we are sure that the eye is not going to go blind because we have missed something then we can consider the possible explanations for other apparent malfunctions at our leisure.

An eye at risk is one that suffers progressive disease without producing warning symptoms. Such an eye may have:

1. creeping field loss due to:
   a. a raised intraocular pressure – commonly
   b. an enlarging pituitary gland – much less commonly
2. A shallow anterior chamber trembling on the brink of acute angle closure.

These are the hallmarks of an eye in danger. They will not be found unless we look for them. The only way to look for them is to carry out the same examination system every time, no matter what the patient complains of. If the ritual does not tell exactly what is wrong, it will tell without ambiguity what is not wrong.

If the field is full, the anterior chamber deep and the intraocular pressure normal, then the eye is safe. It will not go blind because we have missed something that the patient would not know about. If we have missed anything else, we can be sure the patient will tell us.

But if we miss the field loss and miss the shallow anterior chamber and miss the raised pressure, it does not matter how well we treat anything else because in time there will be no functioning eye left to appreciate it.

5. Iritis – a common process in a special organ

The greatest obstacle to medical learning is the firm belief held by every specialty that it is unique. A deep sense of independence sets them all apart and a highly complex patois makes sure they never come together.

In the garish tapestry of sovereign remedies, traditions, eponyms and specifics, the common thread that binds them together is lost. But more things are alike than not. Physiology goes wrong; patients complain; someone with special knowledge interferes and the only difference is where it all happens.

There are only a few processes in pathology: it is the many local variations that make them seem different. Congenital, hereditary, traumatic, neoplastic and so on – the roll call of causation exists for any body tissue. Regional differences do not alter the fundamentals.

Nothing could be more fundamental than inflammation. Whatever its site, it will give rise to:

1. redness – *rubor*
2. heat – *calor*
3. pain – *dolor*
4. swelling – *tumor*
5. loss of function (no Latin tag would be recognizable today).

The visitations do not always follow the sequence below in order but they can:

1. vanish
2. leave adhesions
3. smoulder, replacing special tissue with fibrous tissue
4. involve and damage adjacent structures.

Being in the iris, iritis is of course an ophthalmic problem, but it is still inflammation.

The clinical features can be worked out by reason and a system of management constructed on principles that are not unique to the eye.

The secret is to know without hesitation the essential symptoms and the essential signs. We can follow these landmarks in sequence from first relevant symptom to last sign, through any pathological process. At the end, there will emerge a complete description of the clinical features, a grasp of the problem and a rational notion of how to tackle it.

Since we are dealing with a pathological process, it modifies in time from:

— *acute* to *chronic*

and management modifies from:

— *short term* to *long term*.

Applying this approach to the eye, we might come up with something like this:

1. spasm of the iris muscle produces pain and because the eye is inflamed it will feel hot – *dolor* and *calor*
2. iritis is one of the major causes of a red eye – *rubor*
3. exudation liberates protein and cells into aqueous which appear as floaters in the vision – *tumor* and loss of function
4. the eye may sometimes water and sometimes it may not.

Ophthalmic symptoms always fall prey to classifiers who would subdivide them into mild, moderate and severe. Permutations are then graded into boxed columns of clinical features and the correct diagnoses are meant to roll out the other end like cars from an assembly line.

Were we to point out that what is severe to a hysteric might be trivial to a stoic, we would run the greater risk of having hysteria and stoicism themselves instantly classified into mild, moderate and severe – and possibly very severe, and the diagnostic boxes triumphantly extended.

Of course no action of any consequence is ever taken on the basis of such flimsy subdivisions but they are solemnly learned by heart at the expense of information that might well have been useful. They pass from textbook to textbook where they ferment in the memory along with a whole lot of other pointless trivia and bubble up just in time to turn a firm decision into a cluster of hesitant alternatives.

The seven signs in action

1. *Central vision – distance*: may be blunted.
2. *Central vision* – near: the smallest print may be seen with or without a struggle.

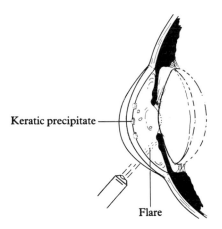

Fig. 5.1 Inflammatory debris, flung out of solution, coats the back of the cornea and may be the only sign of iritis in a mildly inflamed eye. Such deposits are called keratic precipitates. Inflammatory exudate is not optically clear and can be picked up by a fine torch, as is dust or smoke by a projector beam.

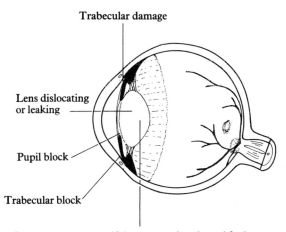

Fig. 5.2 Acute inflammation may silt the trabecular meshwork. Chronic inflammation may damage it with adhesions or block the pupil by the same mechanism.

3. *Field vision*: no reason for constriction.
4. *Cornea*: epithelium no reason to be anything but clear.
    Inflammatory debris sometimes flung up like flotsam by the
    tide on to deep surface of cornea where slight magnification
    reveals it as a series of little white dots.
5. *Pupil*: small and spastic unless irregular from adhesions of
    previous attack – or already dilated by patient who knows
    what happened last time.
6. *Anterior chamber*: no reason to be shallow; protein-rich
    aqueous, not optically clear – will pick up the beam of a
    focusing torch as smoke and dust particles pick up the
    projection beam in a cinema.
7. *Intraocular pressure*: inflammation is an ongoing process. If not
    severe it may have no effect on pressure; however if it is going
    to raise the pressure it will do so in two ways:
    a. it may clog trabecular meshwork – sudden rise of pressure
    b. it may block pupil with adhesions – gradual rise of
       pressure.

MANAGEMENT

The scheme of management is the same whatever organ is
involved. If lack of experience makes us hesitate to do what seems
logical, then that is understandable. It is well to remember that
medical advance has frequently been the product of logic per-
sisting in the face of orthodox derision. It requires great courage
to hold to a new belief when laughter greets every demonstration
of its wisdom.

There was Hickman, the Shropshire veterinarian, who dared
suggest that surgery might be more congenial were the patients
asleep, especially if they could be wakened up again. His successful demonstration of this on a cow did not bring a trail of admir-
ers to his door.

And Semmelweiss, the Viennese accoucheur, not just ignored
but reviled, lost his reason when colleagues refused to believe that
the reduced death rate following childbirth in his wards had
something to do with antiseptics and water and something so
revolutionary as washing the hands.

The follies of history affect us all because, although technology
changes, human nature does not. Medical techniques may

become history as new techniques supplant them, but the principles of management which are common to all branches of medicine never disappear into history because they are eternal.

Although eternal, they are however not ethereal and they can easily split up into practical guidelines. These guidelines progress from:

— *medical* to *surgical*

and from:

— *short term* to *long term.*

Short term

1. The exciting cause should be identified and removed if possible.
2. If the exciting cause is not known then its effects must be curbed if possible.
3. Complications should be anticipated; it should be remembered that remedies frequently have complications also.
4. There is a patient attached to the diseased eye who is in need of sympathy, comfort, reassurance and possibly analgesics.
5. Restoration of function is hopefully the end product of therapeutic intervention.

Long term

The only difference from urgent aims is that the balance of treatment now inclines towards restoration of function after the drama of an acute illness is no longer absorbing all our attention.

Short term

Although iritis may be associated with conditions like ankylosing spondylitis or the collagen disorders, the exact cause of the inflammation is usually not known. Even if we do not know why it has happened iritis is still iritis and we recognize it as such.

If the iritis is secondary to keratitis, the state of the cornea will tell us so.

If it is secondary to acute angle closure the state of the pupil and the depth of the anterior chamber will tell us so.

Suppression of inflammation

If the condition is simply iritis secondary to nothing obvious then topical corticosteroids may be used, to suppress the inflammation and to prevent adhesions forming between the iris and the lens. The frequency of dosage must be tailored to the severity of the condition. Four times daily to the eye has acquired an almost Biblical sanctity, but in many cases, every hour is sometimes not enough.

Dilatation of the pupil

If the iris is going to stick to the lens anyway, despite corticosteroids, then we must at least put some obstacles in the way. The diameter of the pupil can be increased and thick adhesions which would have totally occluded the small pupil might leave gaps if stuck around a larger pupil – and through these gaps, the aqueous will continue to flow.

The eye has much more chance of seeing through a dilated pupil than through a small one plastered with inflammatory debris.

Therefore the pupil must be dilated with some suitable agent. Atropine drops are time-honoured and long-acting. They acquired their name of belladonna from their effect on the ladies of ancient Rome who added lustre to their eyes by dilating their pupils. Black limpid pools beneath tremulous lashes were considered very seductive. This was probably true and for the ladies, the loss of near focus had the matchless advantage of blurring away the deformities of their more mis-shapen consorts.

Intraocular pressure

If the flow of aqueous has been disturbed, then the rise of intraocular pressure has to be controlled. This can be done in two ways:

1. the inflow can be reduced
2. the outflow can be increased.

Topical medications involving beta blockers, or by curious paradox adrenaline, can influence both the inflow and the outflow of aqueous sufficiently to make the pressure safe.

Acetazolamide, a carbonic anhydrase inhibitor, can only be given by mouth at the moment, but topical preparations are under examination. It reduces the production of aqueous by the ciliary epithelium, but also affects the production of bicarbonate in the renal tubules.

It is part of natural law that drugs with good direct effects invariably have bad side effects and we must remember that topical corticosteroids can raise the intraocular pressure in their own right.

In the short term, perfect function is not a top priority but it should be remembered that the patient will want to see again later. Analgesics possibly and assurance certainly will be required, because all patients have an unspoken fear of going blind.

There is generally no short term surgical management.

Long term

If the inflammation continues despite vigorous management we have to balance the dangers to the eye of stopping treatment altogether against the toxic effects from continued medication.

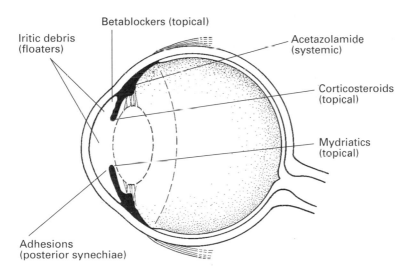

Fig. 5.3   Correct diagnosis based on the essential symptoms and the essential signs is followed by rational treatment based on the essential principles of management.

Long term dosage with corticosteroids may be as damaging to the eye as is the disease itself. If the iritis poisons the aqueous so may the corticosteroid and the lens will make its customary solitary response by going opaque.

Intraocular pressure

If the pressure of the eye remains high following an attack of iritis, then we will have to keep it under control with long term antiglaucoma therapy. Long term administration of acetazolamide can produce metabolic acidosis, renal calculi, finger tingling and a host of related disturbances, all of which should be a reminder of the potential poisons we introduce in the interests of good health.

Long term surgical management

If the aqueous cannot pass through the pupil then it can pass through a hole cut in the peripheral iris – peripheral iridectomy. The iris never heals over these perforations, possibly because of its continued immersion in fluid.

If the trabecular meshwork is itself damaged, the aqueous has to bypass that and drain out of the eye through a surgical fistula into the subconjunctival space.

Should the lens have succumbed either to the disease or to the treatment, then the eye will fail as an organ of vision. Such failure may lead us to consider cataract extraction but it must not be forgotten that any surgery to deal with the sequelae of an old inflammation may place the eye in the grip of a new inflammation.

SUMMARY

Acute inflammation is marked by:

— *rubor*
— *calor*
— *dolor*
— *tumor*
— loss of function.

Chronicity tempers the first four, but may augment the last with fibrosis and adhesion.

Acute iritis and chronic iritis, like any other inflammation, are characterized by all the above and the only qualifying factor is the eye. A history based on the five essential symptoms will lead us to consider the possibility of iritis.

By working our way through the seven essential signs we can recognize that the patient has a red eye and that this red eye is not due to:

1. conjunctivitis
2. keratitis
3. acute angle closure.

There is a danger in standard textbook descriptions that we imagine all diseases occur in their most florid form. Reality is more often an unremarkable onset with the condition gathering momentum and as it goes along, losing its fire in a grumbling destruction of function.

We must use the signs to find what is there and not to fit a model description with symptoms classified in boxes augmented with plus signs. If we see what is there we are then in a position to reverse it again in a logical rational way with our therapeutic actions based on an ordered system of management:

1. medical – short term
            long term
2. surgical – short term
            long term.

With that system we aim to:

1. remove the cause
2. alleviate the ill effects of the cause
3. relieve discomfort
4. restore function.

Together, then, the symptoms, the signs and the management make up a frame around which the description, diagnosis and treatment of any condition can be woven every time by reason and not by rote.

The system must be grooved like a golf swing so that it can function beyond conscious thought when stress and anxiety are conspiring to paralyse the brain with sheer terror. There are other benefits. First of all there is no fear that anything of consequence might be missed. Second, a similar approach can be applied to any system throughout the body. Third, the thoughts released by freedom from fear may be great, may be productive and certainly will be the better for having the whole mind to play with.

6. The red eye

Before we can call an eye abnormal and red, we must first be sure what we mean by normal and white. Such a definition is based on the conjunctival appearances which depend on what lies underneath. To begin with there is the sclera, seen as egg-shell white through the translucent vascular conjunctiva.

The sclera's dominance fades as the conjunctiva folds away into the fornix and then towards the front again, where it becomes pinker and pinker, until it arrives at the deep surface of the lids where a meshwork of deep blood vessels makes the natural appearance quite red.

THREE SERIOUS CAUSES

So much for the normal; there is barely more to the abnormal, for there are only three causes of inflammation that can be called serious, and they all have the same sign – inflammation dominant around the corneo-scleral limbus

At the limbus the vessels connect with those deep inside the eye. If the deep ones dilate as a result of serious inflammation, then these visible vessels dilate also. This so-called corneo-scleral, limbal or ciliary injection is therefore the warning sign that we could be dealing with one of the major three red eyes:

1. keratitis
2. iritis
3. acute angle closure (also known as acute glaucoma).

If the inflammation does not dominate around the corneo-scleral limbus, then we are not dealing with one of the major three.

No textbook is considered complete unless it attempts to distinguish at length every cause of the red eye from every other cause. The upshot is that the baffled reader emerges certain that the eye is red but not too sure of anything else.

There is only one decision to make about a red eye: is it one of the major three or not?

If it is then the basic seven signs carried out in the same way every time will indicate which of the major three it is every time. If it is not one of the major three then it is one of the others and may

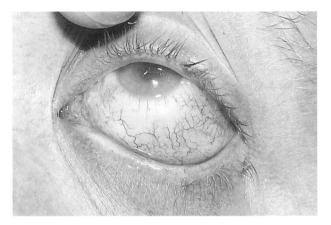

Fig. 6.1   Ciliary injection – the major sign of a serious red eye – in this case due to keratitis, recognised from the broken epithelium. The injection need not be florid.

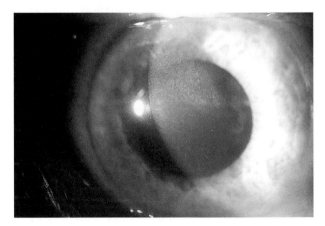

Fig. 6.2   Corneal abrasion. Anything which dislodges the surface epithelium produces a classic area which stains green with fluorescein. The knee-jerk reflex is to apply a topical antibiotic but the quickest cure will be brought about by tape closure.

be managed at leisure in the certainty that no undetected disorder is nibbling away at the more important elements of the eye.

The dominant symptoms of all three are:

— pain
— redness
— watering
— some disturbance of vision.

If the symptoms are florid, as they usually are, we can rarely hope to found any diagnostic distinctions on symptoms alone. Those diagnostic boxes crisscrossed with plus signs only add something else inexplicable to circumstances that are already mysterious enough.

KERATITIS

The positive findings from the seven signs

1. & 2.   *Central vision*: reduction for *distance* and *near*, depending upon actual position of ulcer.
4.   *Cornea*: lustre lost; exact area of deficient epithelium demonstrated with fluorescein.

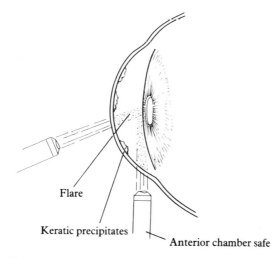

Flare

Keratic precipitates

Anterior chamber safe

Fig. 6.3   Iritis is the least dramatic of the serious red eyes. There is debris on the deep corneal surface and anterior chamber flare. The anterior chamber is safe (eclipse test negative). Intraocular pressure may be raised if the pupil is adherent to the lens or if the drainage meshwork is clogged.

IRITIS

The positive findings from the seven signs

1. & 2. *Central vision – distance* and *near*: anything from normal downwards.

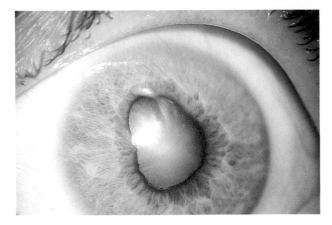

Fig. 6.4 Acute iritis – one of the three serious red eyes. The redness is not always severe enough to be taken seriously. Inflammatory adhesions may develop between the iris and the lens, where they are given the name of posterior synechiae.

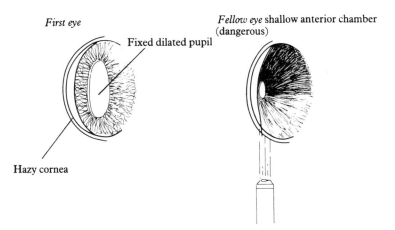

Fig. 6.5 Acute angle closure is one of the three serious red eyes. The cornea is hazy, the pupil fixed and dilated. The anterior chamber is shallow in each eye (eclipse test positive) and the intraocular pressure is grossly raised in the affected eye.

4. *Cornea*: clear; deposits of inflammatory material (keratic precipitates) detectable on deep surface of cornea with magnifying glass.
5. *Pupil*: spastic, unless distorted by previous adhesions or dilated with atropine.
6. *Anterior chamber*: aqueous flare in the affected eye.
7. *Intraocular pressure*: elevation, if present, is not generally main feature.

ACUTE ANGLE CLOSURE

The evident distress of the patient usually cuts short any addition to the history of

1. haloes
2. frontal headache
3. transient attacks of blurred vision at dusk.

The positive findings from the seven signs

1. & 2. *Central vision – distance* and *near*: grievously affected.
4. *Cornea*: steamy and oedematous – deeper signs obscured.
5. *Pupil* – if seen: fixed and dilated.

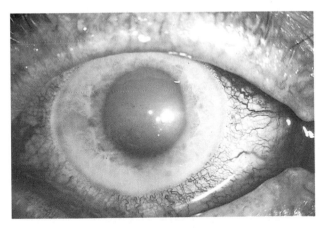

Fig. 6.6 Acute angle closure – one of the three serious red eyes. Inflammation is dominant around the corneoscleral limbus. The pupil is fixed and dilated. The anterior chamber is shallow.

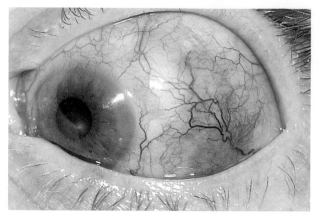

Fig. 6.7   Scleritis. This might be considered the fourth serious red eye but is a rarity compared with the other three. Inflammation of collagen, often at a systemic level, produces atrophy of the sclera allowing the deeper structures to be seen either as black rounded elevations through the sclera or as black fragments rupturing the sclera.

6.   *Anterior chamber*: shallow in both eyes; if obscured on affected side, eclipse test on fellow eye will leave iris remote from light in shadow.

7.   *Intraocular pressure*: affected eye rock hard; acutely tender.

Once we can recognize when an eye is inflamed by one of the major three we will also be in a position to recognize when it is not. As a general rule, the less dangerous a red eye is the more alarming it will appear. Subconjunctival haemorrhage and conjunctivitis can both seem fearful and if the cardinal signs of the cornea, the pupil, the anterior chamber and the intraocular pressure are neglected in favour of the overall impression, then this impression may be given a greater significance than it deserves.

SUMMARY

Of the three major red eyes

1.   *Acute angle closure* has the most signs:
      — diminished vision
      — hazy cornea

— dilated pupil
— shallow anterior chamber
— raised intraocular pressure.
2. *Keratitis* – the dominant feature is a broken corneal epithelium.
3. *Iritis* may have only ciliary injection to mark it off from other lesser causes of a red eye. Very close examination will reveal white deposits on deep surface of cornea (keratic precipitates). A spastic pupil is possible.

The deep vessels connect with their tributaries on the scleral surface from the corneal edge to the rectus insertions. They are seen through the conjunctiva and seen most clearly beside the corneal margin where the conjunctiva is most tightly adherent.

The unchanging guide is to use the same seven signs every time and not to take flight from reason just because someone's triad or someone else's tetrad does not come instantly to mind.

7. Common disorders of the outer eye

The outer eye is an alliance – a coalition of partners linked together for their mutual benefit. Their association is not unlike that of the EEC.

Outside, we have Holland represented by the eyelids – on the fringe of Europe, keeping danger out and protecting vital structures within.

The conjunctiva can only be France – with her shadowy folds and tendency to become inflamed from time to time.

The cornea – important, round, smooth and transparent – has to be Germany.

Whilst Britain – all tearful nostalgia for when the world was young – can have no serious rivals as the lacrimal gland.

The outer eye is a moist structure and like the mouth it is most comfortable when shut. Also like the mouth, it has to open from time to time. Because of this, its entire arrangement allows the eye to experience, when open, the comfort it enjoys when shut – provided that it does not stay open for too long.

The cornea is not totally without its own protection: it senses pain to a degree achieved by few other tissues. But, once it has registered pain, it has exhausted its repertoire of defence and relies on the other three.

The eyelashes, like cat's whiskers, trigger reflex closure of the lids when touched. In addition, their continued blinking of the lids spreads tears over the cornea, clearing away debris and producing optical perfection.

The conjunctival folds are not at all superfluous. They allow free movement of the eye, the conjunctival glands contribute fat and mucous to the tears, and indeed without a conjunctiva the eye cannot exist as an organ of vision.

The tear gland provides the essential moisture without which the eye would dry out to the point of uselessness.

Although patients will draw attention to malfunction of the outer eye, we must remember that there is also an internal eye which they may not think worthy of any attention and which may be the site of an even greater malfunction. To ignore the inner eye is to be like first class passengers on a sinking liner, taking comfort that the leak is in the tourist section.

This means that whatever the complaint we must 'think aqueous' and go through the seven signs which direct us to find appearances that are relevant both to the outer and the inner eye.

Inflammation, particularly of the lash roots and of the conjunctiva, does not always respond to what we have to offer as treatment. The continued failure of our medications will torment us with uncertainties. The seven signs must be our guide. Although they may not always tell us what is wrong they will always tell us what is not wrong.

If

1. the vision is unaffected
2. the cornea clear
3. the pupil normal
4. the anterior chamber safe
5. the pressure acceptable

then the eye is not going to go blind for unsuspected and undetected reasons whilst we are grappling unsuccessfully with unconnected problems.

A complete list of possible external malfunctions would fill a book twice this size and only those of the sternest character could read it with any sense of improving discomfort. Disorders of the outer eye are usually obvious, since they usually entail some deviation from a normal state that we see every day every time we look at a face, and we do not need a book to know what one looks like. The seven signs will allow us to elaborate a rational form of management.

Complaints of irritation, pain, redness and change of appearance are generally too diffuse to be of any locating value. This should be no obstacle to diagnosis because:

1. the part to blame is usually obvious
2. if other members of the alliance are affected also, that should be obvious also
3. we have to go through the seven signs anyway.

MALPOSITION OF THE EYELIDS

Ectropion

The lower lid, under the influence of time, may droop from the eye, rather like that of a bloodhound. A facial palsy may produce the same appearance. A contracting scar makes the separation more unyielding and a laceration, tearing the lid margin, drops the lid into two separate halves.

Resultant malfunction

1. The lacrimal punctum can no longer pick up tears – the eye waters.
2. Exposure – drying conjunctiva turns to skin.
    – drying cornea is prepared to exchange clarity for survival.

Action

1. Reverse exposure.
2. Deal with consequences of exposure.

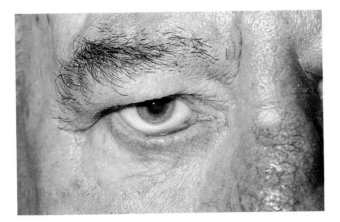

Fig. 7.1   Ectropion – a breach in the alliance of the external eye. The cornea is exposed. The eye waters and the palpable conjunctiva turns to skin.

Short term (medical):

1. Topical lubrication – artificial tears replace loss from evaporation.
2. Closure of the eyelids with adhesive tape unambiguously terminates the exposure, at least for a short time.

Long term (surgical): The cure is removal of a wedge of eyelid, to shorten the lid and so to replace it against the eyeball.

Entropion

Age may also turn the eyelid inwards.

Resultant malfunction

1. Excoriation of the cornea – the lashes work against the epithelium like a scrubbing brush.
2. Actual corneal infection.

Action

Short term (medical):

1. The lid can be turned outwards with tape adhering to the skin from the lash margin to the cheek.

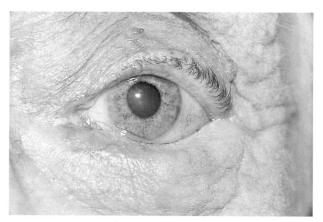

Fig. 7.2   Entropion. The lower lid turns inwards, abrading the corneal surface with the eyelashes.

2.   Irritation soothed with artificial tears.
3.   Infection countered with intensive topical antibiotics.

Long term (surgical):

1.   Chromic catgut from the lower edge of the tarsal plate
     outwards and upwards through the eyelid to below the lash
     line (Snellen's sutures) induces scar tissue which turns the
     eyelid outwards again.
     18 months later the manoeuvre may have to be repeated but
     it has the advantage that it can be repeated and does not
     mutilate the lid in the process.
2.   Splitting and wedge resection of the lower lid.
     A more complicated stratagem (Fould's procedure) turns the
     lid outwards more definitely but with greater surgical
     discomfort.

TRICHIASIS

Lashes pointing in the wrong direction can destroy the cornea.
The condition behaves like entropion, except that the lid does not
turn in.

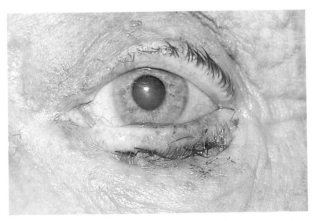

Fig. 7.3   Entropion treated with Snellen's sutures, strands of chromic catgut
stitched from the inner surface of the lid to beneath the lash margin.

Action

Short term: Any ocular ointment can protect the cornea. The lashes may be plucked out only to return later with renewed vigour.

Long term: Electrolysis down each hair follicle offers still the best definitive alternative to epilation.

If there are too many lashes, then all the patience in the world will not direct a needle down each one. The lash line has to be turned away from the eye in a plastic reconstruction, sometimes requiring a fragment of mucous membrane from the mouth to take on the role of conjunctiva.

BLEPHARITIS

In its simple form this is essentially dandruff of the eyelashes. A more severe ulcerative form is a destructive inflammation which involves the adjacent skin as well. The flecks that cluster round the base of the lashes have to be washed away with warm water before anything useful can be applied.

Action

The most useful application is an antibiotic ointment – rubbed deeply into the lash roots, perhaps three times a day for three days at a time. When the scales return, the whole process will have to be started all over again.

THE DRY EYE

A reduced production of tears is the most common cause of:

1. stabbing pains in the eye
2. recurrent conjunctivitis
3. punctate erosions of the corneal epithelium.

Action

Short term: Topical artificial tears seek to replace from a bottle a solution similar to the mucus–lipid–aqueous blend that makes up normal tears.

The frequency of dosage will depend on how dry the eye is, but in extreme conditions tears from a bottle are just not enough.

Long term: A more radical approach is to block one of the outflow canaliculi. Since most of us have abandoned walking on all fours, the upper canaliculus plays a less important role than it does in some monkeys.

The upper duct can be blocked permanently with cautery – an easy manoeuvre, under local anaesthesia.

However before proceeding to that extreme, we can see if blockage is to be of benefit with a temporary plug of gelatine which will melt away after about a week.

In cases of even greater severity, the lower punctum may be similarly blocked, though with much greater caution because it is the major drainage channel from the conjunctival sac.

SUPERFICIAL PUNCTATE KERATITIS

If the corneal epithelium is pitted with multiple erosions, then the diagnosis can be made easily with fluorescein.

Action

In general if the corneal epithelium is absent, the instillation of medications into the conjunctival sac does not always make it grow again. In fact it may do the reverse.

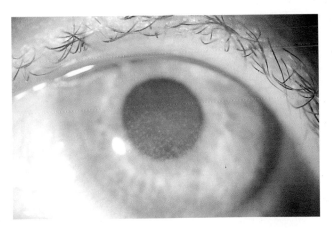

Fig. 7.4 Superficial punctate keratitis – breaking of the choreal epithelium, due either to ultraviolet exposure or grossly deficient tear secretion. Can be visually devastating and painful and responds best to total closure, when the eye is at its most comfortable.

Whilst moistening the eye with artificial tears may reduce the erosions to some degree, the most effective management is to close the eyelids with adhesive tape to give the epithelium time to regenerate in peace before exposing it again to take its chance in the open world.

CONCRETIONS

Concretions are tiny calcareous deposits in the tarsal conjunctiva. It is possible that epithelium, folding on itself, acts as an irritant, which the eyelid like an oyster rolls into a pearl. Unfortunately the pearl is not smooth and may fret against the corneal epithelium, with predictable results.

Action

Concretions may be scraped away with a needle under topical anaesthesia.

SUPERFICIAL FOREIGN BODY

Although patients may present with irritation, their attempts to remove a foreign body may produce quite a degree of pain as well.

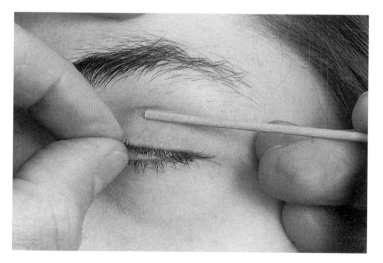

Fig. 7.5 Turning the upper lid. It is always wise to tell the patient what you are trying to do. For the dextrous the manoeuvre can sometimes be achieved without the little stick.

Subtarsal foreign body

All manner of air-borne particles – grit or fragments of an insect – can slip by, before the lashes can trigger the blink reflex.

Enraged and futile attempts to rub them out of the eye can actually produce greater damage than the offending particle might have managed on its own.

Action

The lower lid can be easily pulled open. The upper lid is another matter.

It can be everted by pulling on the lashes whilst pressing the upper margin of the tarsal plate against the eye.

If the foreign body is up in the fornix, that too can be brought into view by pressing the lower lid firmly against the eye.

A drop of local anaesthetic might make the search and subsequent removal a little less unpleasant.

Corneal foreign body

Although the blink reflex, triggered by the cat's whisker eyelashes, keeps the cornea free from larger particles, smaller ones can

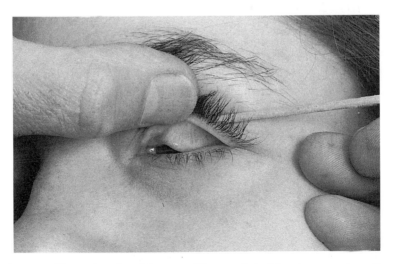

Fig. 7.6   The conjunctiva of the upper lid exposed. At this point, pressure on the lower lid can bring the upper conjunctival fornix into view.

sometimes slip in unnoticed. They lodge on the corneal epithelium and then resist all attempts by the lids to blink them away. Various manoeuvres can succeed where the lids failed, but not before a topical anaesthetic, like benoxinate (oxybuprocaine), is applied.

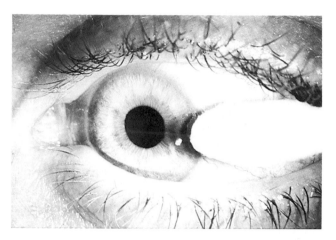

Fig. 7.7 Superficial corneal foreign bodies are not uncommon. Removal should be tried at first with a cotton bud, but only after the application of topical anaesthetic.

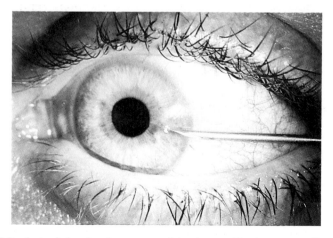

Fig. 7.8 A steady hand and some sort of simple magnification can get direct removal of the foreign body with a needle when a cotton bud has failed.

We should try first with a moistened cotton-tipped applicator, moving thereafter to a disposable needle. The corneal spud – a blunt edged foreign body remover, as delicate as a hoof – seems designed to remove corneal epithelium whilst leaving the foreign body undisturbed.

TARSAL CYST

When a stagnant tarsal gland becomes infected, it turns into a meibomian abscess. When the infection has gone, the cyst hardens into a small lump (chalazion) which, if large enough, will distort vision.

Resultant malfunction

Acute: a painful inflammatory lump, leaking pus from the inner surface of the eyelid.
   Chronic: a vision-disturbing lump.

Action

Short term (medical):

1. Intensive topical antibiotics may bring about complete resolution.
2. Heat in one form or another can certainly produce comfort and may speed the resolution. A wooden spoon wrapped in

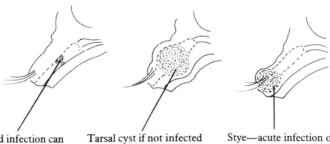

Tarsal gland infection can be aborted early stage   Tarsal cyst if not infected requires curettage   Stye—acute infection of lash root

Fig. 7.9   A blocked tarsal gland can be infected and the start of a series. Infection of the lash root lies nearer the lid margin than does an infected cyst. The first may be mistaken for the second and both may be treated with intensive antibiotics and heat. Repeated infections might well indicate a systemic disturbance like diabetes.

hot wet lint is traditional. The lower rim of a hot tea cup is possibly more convenient.

Long term (surgical): If resolution is incomplete, the resultant cyst has to be incised on the deep surface of the eyelid.

One infected cyst may be the first of a series which can be aborted by timely topical antibiotics started at the first hint of a symptom and continued for some days after the pain is gone.

STYE

An infected lash root appears to the unobservant as an infected tarsal cyst and vice versa.

Action

Short term (medical): Treatment in the acute phase is identical to that for a tarsal cyst. The only real practical difference is that a stye will not end up as a chalazion.

Long term (medical): Recurrent infections in the eyelids can sometimes be an indication of some underlying condition – like diabetes.

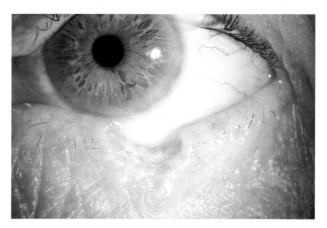

Fig. 7.10   Rodent ulcer. Hardened, rolled edges of a lesion that never seems to get better are the classic signs of this condition. Here it is seen living up to its name, nibbling away mercilessly at the eyelid but as yet, curiously, with no major effect on the cornea.

RODENT ULCER

Also known as basal cell carcinoma, this most common tumour of the eyelids presents as a dimpled lump with rolled edges and apparently always in the grip of some indolent or recurrent infection from which it never seems to escape.

Resultant malfunction

It is not called rodent ulcer for nothing and has the potential to nibble away to extinction all adjacent structures.

Action

Radiotherapy offers as much hope of success as does complete surgical excision and with considerably less discomfort. However, with both methods we have to remember the possibility of damage to the lacrimal puncta and canaliculi and, in the upper lid particularly, radiotherapy threatens permanent obstruction of the tiny ducts carrying tears from the gland into the upper conjunctival fornix.

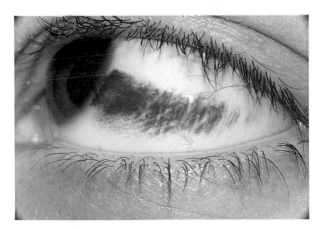

Fig. 7.11   Subconjunctival haemorrhage – a dramatic appearance causing much needless anxiety. The secret is to recognise that: 1) the vision is unimpaired; 2) the cornea, pupil and anterior chamber are normal; 3) the intraocular pressure is within acceptable limits.

SUBCONJUNCTIVAL HAEMORRHAGE

Because of the normal appearances of the normal conjunctiva, the sudden presence of blood scattered over a wide area can terrify both the patient and the doctor into a diagnosis of something appalling.

Although usually described as painless, the condition does bring with it a slight dragging sensation, but nothing more.

It is recognised by the total obliteration of vascular markings and total normality of the seven signs.

When recurrent and bilateral and associated with haemorrhages elsewhere, any bleeding tendency must be investigated. Haemorrhage harmless in the conjunctiva could have the most fearful effects within the eye or within the brain.

Resultant malfunction

None.

Action

Investigation as and when indicated.

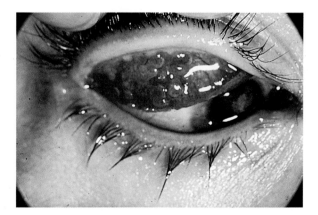

Fig. 7.12   Spring catarrh – one cause of giant papillae on the palpebral conjunctiva. The lid, instead of protecting the eye, works over it like a scrubbing brush.

SPRING CATARRH

An allergic condition, spring catarrh begins in early life and tends to improve during the mid-teens. More common perhaps in those children unhappy enough to suffer from eczema and asthma, it produces joint papillae on the deep surface of the eyelids, threatening the cornea and indeed occasionally abrading it into an ulcer.

As the asthma and eczema fade away, so does the spring catarrh. Although potentially damaging in its own right, greater damage comes from dirty fingernails insinuated beneath the eyelids to scratch away the irritation.

Resultant malfunction

1. An irritable red eye.
2. The scrubbing-brush effect of the eyelid on the corneal surface.

Action

Sodium cromoglycate, happily without side effects and unhappily sometimes without any effect, may safely eliminate symptoms and signs.

Topical corticosteroids, however, are most likely to curb the exuberance of the conjunctival papillae. Their use has to be monitored because on their own account they may offer, in exchange for exuberant papillae, an exuberant intraocular pressure.

Once the epithelium is broken, a bandage contact lens can keep the papillae at bay while the corneal epithelium heals itself.

CORNEAL ULCER

From a practical point of view the commonest danger is a simple breach of the corneal epithelium due either to trauma, infection or some suspension of the protective alliance like ectropion or tear deficiency.

Any breach of the corneal epithelium is given the name keratitis.

HERPES SIMPLEX (DENDRITIC ULCER)

Though probably less common than bacterial infection and for some reason possibly less common nowadays, this viral invasion can bring with it both short-term and long-term damage.

Emerging from its fastness in the trigeminal ganglion, the virus can select its victim at random. If it chooses the cornea, the classic branching figure, with its dendritic pattern highlighted with fluorescein, can neither be mistaken or forgotten.

As with any other infection, it may not stay where it starts but seeds itself across the corneal epithelium penetrating the stroma through Bowman's membrane, trailing in its wake the inevitable scar.

Resultant malfunction

1. Pain.
2. Visual defect which may become permanent.
3. Loss of pain sensation in the cornea.

Action

Short term: The drug of choice nowadays is acyclovir. It is prepared as an ointment — 3% w/w in a white soft paraffin base.

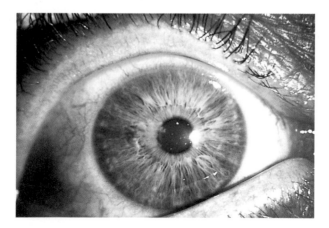

Fig. 7.13 Dendritic ulcer – keratitis – one of the three serious red eyes. Ciliary injection is not marked. A small dendritic figure is seen outlined in green with fluorescein.

has a selective toxicity in that it inhibits virus replication without inhibiting replication of the host cell.

The ointment should be placed within the lower conjunctival sac five times a day and treatment should be continued for some days after healing is apparent.

Acyclovir has now virtually eclipsed the other antivirals and five times a day is not a tentative addition to the scriptural dosage of four times a day. It is a requirement brought about by the pharmacological nature of the drug.

Long term: Even after the virus has been destroyed, the corneal epithelium may still remain broken. No drug can make it heal. It will regenerate in its own good time beneath closed eyelids. In the shorter term this may be achieved with adhesive tape. In the longer term it may be necessary to stitch the eyelids together (tarsorrhaphy).

The virus, however, permanently destroys pain sensation in the cornea, thus destroying the cornea's only defence mechanism. Tape closure from time to time, almost like a transient prophylactic tarsorrhaphy, can sometimes help the cornea to resist future invasion.

BACTERIAL ULCER

Corneal laceration or perforation is a perfect entry port for any pathogenic organism which happens to be in the vicinity. An abscess, a white fluffy cotton-wool-like opacity, forms in the corneal stroma and if aggressive may seep into the eye to form a fluid level in the anterior chamber – like a white hyphaema.

Resultant malfunction

1. Infection threatens the whole eye (endophthalmitis).
2. Permanent loss of clarity.

Action

Short term:
1. Intensive application of topical antibiotics – usually chloramphenicol.
2. Systemic medication with flucloxacillin if *Staphylococcus aureus* is thought to be the cause, together with ampicillin for

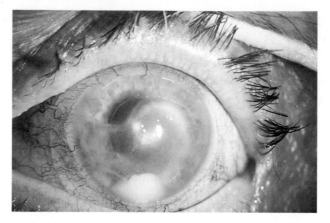

Fig. 7.14 Hypopyon. A collection of white pus in the anterior chamber indicates severe intraocular inflammation and possible infection. The cornea has clearly been damaged. The pupil is dilated, possibly from bi-mydriatics, and the redness around the corneoscleral limbus is what we would expect in the presence of active inflammation.

all the rest. In practice, both tend to be given, at a dosage of 250 mg four times daily.

3. Antibiotic can also be delivered by injection beneath the conjunctiva, possibly relieving infection but bringing with it intense pain.

4. Topical mydratics like atropine will be given for reasons already explained in Chapter 5.

Long term: If scars develop following either viral or bacterial infection, then eventually the only treatment may be a corneal graft. The cornea accepts the graft more happily than other tissues because it has no blood vessels. Unfortunately, corneal ulcers tend to produce abnormal blood vessels which carry with them rejecting antibodies.

CORNEAL EROSION

Should the epithelium be dislodged from its connection with Bowman's membrane, as it may be following simple injuries, it adheres overnight instead to the eyelid which, on opening, tears it away from the eye. The pain is fearful and when the patient has recovered, after a few days the whole cycle may begin again. The accident is found frequently in mothers gazing in admiration at their little bundles, from whom the last thing they expect is a punch in the eye.

Resultant malfunction

1. Pain.
2. Recurrence.

Action

Short term: No topical medications can make the corneal epithelium grow again. Tape closure is the only way to allow the breach to heal.

Long term: Once the eye has healed, some lubricant such as topical castor oil should be instilled nightly to prevent adhesion between the eyelid and the corneal epithelium. Long term does not mean a week, and 6 months would not be unusual.

SATURDAY NIGHT EYE (NOCTURNAL LAGOPHTHALMOS)

When the evening festivities have given way to deep slumber, the morning headache is sometimes further complicated by fierce pain when the eyes appear to open. The problem is that they have not been fully closed overnight. Dehydration of the epithelium coupled with general body dehydration causes exquisite agony when the capacity for sensation returns and the eyes open further to discover what happened the night before.

Action

As for corneal erosion.

CORNEAL LACERATION

As can be guessed, the danger is one of infection and damage to the delicate lens and aqueous drainage apparatus. It must be remembered that what went in might not have come out again and a retained intraocular foreign body will eventually destroy the eye by infection or by the deposition of metallic salts throughout its vital tissues.

Resultant malfunction

The laceration is
1. A perfect entry portal for infection.
2. A perfect exit portal for ocular contents should any pressure be applied carelessly to the globe.

Action

Short term:

1. Diagnose what has happened.
2. Topical antibiotics and a pad are probably the safest first aid measure prior to referral to hospital.

PTERYGIUM

A degenerative accumulation of tissue in the deep layers of the conjunctiva, occurring along the line of the opening eyelids. More common perhaps in Europeans living in tropical exile, the condition is benign until it threatens to move across the cornea. Adopting the form of a wing — hence its name — it may advance relentlessly across the cornea from one side to the other, trailing a scar over the pupil line.

Pterygium is evident in portraits of Admiral Nelson of Trafalgar fame. Indeed, it is likely that it was not as a result of injury at

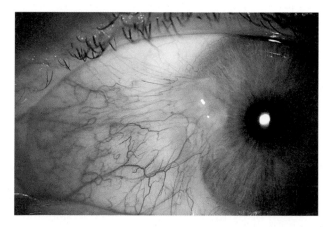

Fig. 7.15   Pterygium. Once the corneal border is crossed and the corneal tissue is violated it will be forever opaque. Removal can only prevent further opacity.

all that one eye was sightless. Rather, a combination of pterygium and presbyopia did more harm to both eyes than the French guns did to one.

Early excision into such a lesion is necessary before it produces a permanent scar. The condition must not be confused with a pinguecula, a flabby yellow nodule which occupies the same area of conjunctiva but never threatens to cross the corneal frontier.

EPISCLERITIS

A painful inflammatory nodule sometimes associated with rheumatic disorders — but usually not.

Resultant malfunction

1. Pain.
2. The danger of mistaking it for a conjunctivitis. The nodule heaped in one area should give the clue.

Action

Intensive topical corticosteroids.

ROSACEA

Rosacea is a metabolic disturbance which produces blotchy inflammation over the cheeks and nose and may also affect the eyes, producing the same blotchy inflammation in the conjunctiva and tongue-shaped inflammatory advances across the cornea itself.

Resultant malfunction

1. Pain and irritation.
2. Danger of corneal scarring.

Action

Topical corticosteroids take the anger out of acute exacerbations.

In recent years the long-term administration of systemic tetracycline in low dosage has been effective in preventing acute attacks altogether.

A total ban on alcohol, spicy cuisine and other pleasing diversions has been recommended. However, there is no record that colonial administrators sustained on a diet of *burra pegs* and fierce curries had a greater incidence of blotchy faces than did their more abstemious counterparts at home.

HERPES ZOSTER OPHTHALMICUS

This infection by the chickenpox virus (varicella) causes sacculation along any branch of the ophthalmic division of the trigeminal nerve. Vesicles change to pustules and form thick tenacious crusts which appear in crops and sprays over the forehead and upper eyelids.

Any of the tissues supplied by the ophthalmic division can be affected but not always all of them. Whatever happens can easily be worked out by considering first of all the pathological behaviour of the virus — which is well known — and working in sequence through the tissues which may be affected.

Resultant malfunction

In the short term the shingles may produce dermatitis, conjunctivitis, keratitis and iritis. The intraocular pressure may rise as a result of the iritis.

In the long term the skin may be scarred and painful. The conjunctiva tends to escape without untoward sequelae but the cornea deprived by the virus of its pain sensation is liable to break down from time to time into multiple pinpoint erosion.

The pressure may remain elevated and it should not be forgotten that the patient is often in the age group when it is elevated anyway by chronic simple glaucoma.

The iritis may induce a cataract.

Even when all is settled, pain may persist long after the scabs have gone. Shingles has been called 'the girdle of roses from hell'. As far as the eye is concerned, although the word 'girdle' may not be appropriate, its source without doubt is.

Each aspect of this condition is dealt with elsewhere in the book. To construct a diagnosis and management is a salutary exercise to demonstrate how little new information actually needs to be learned. An answer will be found in Chapter 24.

TRACHOMA

Trachoma must be the commonest cause of blindness in the Third World. Ironically, the infective agents — the chlamydiae — do not in themselves destroy vision. They produce a toxin which excites a lymphocytic reaction and scar formation in the subepithelial areas of the conjunctiva. The result is a dry eye which is a fertile breeding ground for secondary invasion.

In countries where water costs more than petrol, soap is not high on the list of priorities and a whole range of bacteria can complicate the primary disease. The inevitable result is scarring everywhere. The lids are distorted, the tear inflow blocked, the cornea infiltrated with blood vessels and the whole external alliance including the sacred cornea is hopelessly disrupted.

Ideally, management should start with prevention, education, the provision of public health facilities and the elimination of filth.

In the acute stages, tetracycline ointment is effective. In the later stages surgery is required to remodel distorted lids, turn the lashes outwards and reconstruct the conjunctival sac. Corneal opacities may respond to corneal grafting if the cornea is not riddled with blood-borne rejecting antibodies.

CORTICOSTEROIDS AND THE EYE

All topical corticosteroids figure prominently amongst ophthalmic preparations. It cannot be said too often that use of these drugs in the presence of the herpes simplex virus may be the first step into the law courts. They have no rivals in their bold contribution to ocular pathology. Yet their frequent prescription is supported by a reason that may trace back into the mists of our undergraduate subconsciousness. The sophistical change may be linked thus:

1. A red eye means inflammation.
2. Inflammation means scars.
3. Scars mean an opaque cornea.
4. Corticosteroids suppress inflammation, will prevent scars and will keep the cornea clear.
5. Therefore corticosteroids must be applied to any red eye.

A fallacious practice which continues to condemn patient to needless and permanent visual loss — hopeful to the end because they feel better as they continue to get worse.

Corticosteroids must never be instilled into the conjunctival sac until sodium fluorescein has proved that the corneal epithelium is intact. Even if it is, corticosteroids have other side effects.

1. Fungal growth flourishes under the protection of prolonged dosage.
2. The systemic effects of water retention are parallelled within the eye. Because the eye is not distensible the intraocular pressure may rise to dangerous levels.
3. Corticosteroids have also been implicated in cataract formation.

SODIUM CROMOGLYCATE

This drug, already with some success to its name in the treatment of asthma and hay fever, has a prophylactic rather than a curative effect. It is believed to prevent the antigen—antibody combination

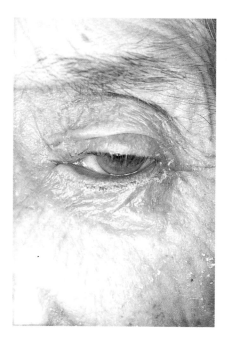

Fig. 7.16 Allergic response. Topical medications share one common feature: their capacity to provoke an allergic inflammation, the behaviour of which does not alter whatever the exciting allergen (which, as often as not, is the preservative).

from disrupting mast cells, thus preventing the release of histamine and similar substances. Although beautifully effective in diagram, with all the potential vasodilators trapped by a defensive ring of chemical formulae, beauty is not always duplicated in life and some subtle inflammatory combination may yet escape from this molecular cordon.

ALLERGIC RESPONSES

Unfortunately, all drugs, even those used to treat allergy, have a capacity to provoke some allergic reaction themselves. Ophthalmic allergies are recognised by swelling of the tarsal conjunctiva and skin and oedema spreading from the lid margin to beyond the orbital limits. As time goes on, the skin takes on a leathery sheen which gives way to superficial flaking. The diagnosis is usually obvious and some cortisone lotion applied only to the skin after the offending application has been stopped will reduce the oedema rapidly and ease the patient's resentment with equal speed.

PTOSIS

When the upper lid fails to rise above the pupil line, the explanation must vary with age, the mode of onset and any associated features.

Children are clearly more likely to have the congenital variety, although adults may just have put up with it for a long time.

Structures that defy gravity in youth tend to droop with age and the upper lid is a classic example.

Both congenital and senile ptosis are characterised by the total absence of sinister symptoms and by any defect in the cranial nerves.

However, the sudden onset of a dropped lid usually means that something has gone wrong with the cranial nerve. A third nerve palsy virtually immobilises the eye, enlarges the pupil and raises the disturbing possibility of an intracranial aneurysm.

A more leisurely onset of a dropped lid may follow some disturbance of the cervical sympathetic chain which innervates the movement of the upper eyelid and pupil. It does not interfere with eye movements, does not enlarge the pupil. In fact it makes it small. It does not prevent voluntary muscles from raising the eyelids, should they be asked to do so.

This collection of signs has been called Horner's syndrome too long for the name to be dropped. The cause is not always malignant. Prolapsed cervical discs and the resulting reparative surgery have been known to produce these signs. Textbooks always mention tumour at the apex of the lung. More rarely, the condition may be congenital, particularly if the iris in the affected eye is a different colour from that of the other side.

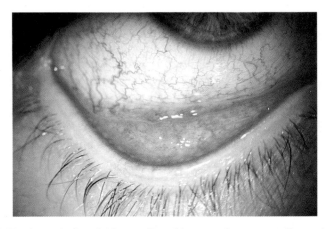

Fig. 7.17   Acute conjunctivitis – confirmed by normal cornea, pupil, anterior chamber and intraocular pressure (unless this is raised for other reasons).

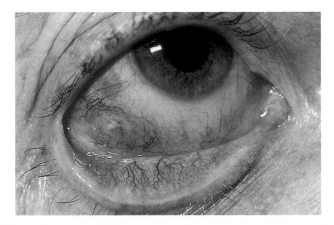

Fig. 7.18   Subconjunctival abscess – potentially dangerous but not one of the three serious red eyes (note the normal cornea, pupil and, presumably, anterior chamber). Possible causes are legion, but an infected stitch or subconjunctival foreign body are the most likely.

CONJUNCTIVITIS

There can be no diagnosis more frequent than conjunctivitis, even when it is actually something else. Now, any inflammation of the conjunctiva is a conjunctivitis secondary to whatever is near enough to be to blame, like a lacerated eyelid or the irritation of a subtarsal foreign body. But redness, dominant in the conjunctiva and not so dominant round the corneo–scleral limbus, and with no obvious exciting condition, is primary conjunctivitis.

The causes of inflammation are legion. Infection does not need to be bacterial. It can range over all the available organisms. And the cause is not always infection. Allergy, chemical irritation, radiation, lack of tears   they can all produce a red eye and a diagnosis of conjunctivitis.

Nonetheless, the most common insult is bacterial infection, aided and abetted not infrequently by tear deficiency.

The worse a red eye looks the less serious it tends to be. Conjunctival infections can look fearful. The important thing is not to suspend our reason just because the inflammation happens to be in the eye. The absence of visual symptoms – and of anything positive from the seven signs, if we only have the courage to go through them – will provide comforting proof that the cause of the complaint lies fairly and squarely in the conjunctiva. The addition of purulent discharge will support that belief.

Action

Short term (medical): Treatment must be intensive topical antibiotics, usually in drop form. The important word is intensive. It is somehow enshrined in the ophthalmic tradition that all drugs have a magical effect if given four times a day. An acute raging conjunctivitis might continue to rage despite topical applications every hour, forcing us into systemic treatment as well.

Of recent years fusidic acid has become available as a sustained release, viscous formulation which can be effective on a twice-daily dosage. The quality must have much to recommend it in patients whose fingers cannot manipulate drop bottles and whose memories prevent them from trying.

Conjunctivitis is not a casual disease. It is extremely painful and always carries the danger of spread into the deeper ocular structures. Although strict practice should demand a statement from the bacteriologists about the organism and the best antibiotic, actual practice usually demands instant action.

Non-purulent conjunctivitis

Such inflammation of the conjunctiva that does not respond to intensive topical therapy can reasonably be ascribed to viral infection. The condition may be isolated or part of an epidemic shared by users of the same swimming pool.

It must not be forgotten, however, that excessive chlorination of the water to prevent such infections may produce conjunctival appearances not dissimilar to the infection they seek to prevent. It must also be remembered that the benzalkonium chloride used to preserve the formulation of all these drugs can in itself produce a not dissimilar appearance which may become worse as yet more preservative-containing drugs are applied to the eye in the hope of making things better. Clearly in such cases preservative-free applications have to be considered, and indeed even stopping all applications may produce a dramatic improvement.

SUMMARY

The external eye is a moist collaboration between three humble structures, each dependent on the other and which together form the rank and file of the Imperial Guard for Her Corneal Clearness.

The tears provide the moisture. The conjuntiva provides the mucus and the lipids which prolong the wetting action of tears thus creating that perfect environment in which the cornea flourishes with such smooth transparency. The eyelids opening and, more to the point, closing, sweep these tears over the corneal surface, granting to the eye when open, the comfort it craves when shut.

Should any one of the three fail in their duty, there are always two results to consider – firstly the direct cause of the failure and secondly the extent to which this failure has weakened the alliance.

As usual, a complete list of causes could be constructed over several pages in the certain knowledge that no-one would be any the wiser for reading it.

The first step to sensible clinical management, then, is not to produce such a causal litany but to recognise that the partners of the alliance are at odds with each other and that the alliance itself has broken down.

The aims and mechanisms of treatment of any disease of any part of the body are founded on principle and order. Once we have identified something wrong, the principle is to try to make it right by eliminating the cause or at least by diminishing its ill effects.

The order is to proceed to total restoration of function by medical means then by surgical means. The short-term goals give way in time to longer-term goals, both the better for not being based on the knee-jerk prescription of antibiotics four times a day every time an eye is red.

8. The watering eye

The eye could not survive without tears, but when something is amiss with the lacrimal system, a wet eye is what people complain most bitterly about. A dry eye, on the other hand, with its associated complications and its potential for greater danger, is inventively ascribed to a variety of causes none of which is usually connected in any way with the lacrimal apparatus.

There are two kinds of tear production. First, the basal flow keeps the external alliance moist. The second, reflex flow is the response to some disturbance – like a foreign body or a finger in the eye.

Should the basal flow be diminished, the ensuing grittiness may stimulate the remaining tear cells into activity. A dry eye therefore sometimes responds to its dryness by watering.

Epiphora

This is the name given to any condition where tears appear on the wrong side of the eyelids. The usual cause is diminished drainage, but a red, irritable eye will water for reasons that do not require an investigation of epiphora.

Drainage

The tear outflow system from the eyelids to the nose depends on open ducts and neat contact between the eyelid and the eyeball. A lacrimal punctum in the wrong position is a commoner cause of watering than is blockage along the actual ducts themselves.

Canalicular block

Loss of patency between the punctum and the tear sac is particularly hard to treat. The tubes are so fine that surgery upon them may increase rather than decrease the obstruction.

Nasolacrimal duct

Children

A membrane at the lower end of the nasolacrimal duct occasionally remains imperforate. It is possible to clear this membrane by probing the duct under general anaesthesia. However, in the absence of lacrimal sac infection there is much to be said for waiting in the hope that simple growth will produce the necessary opening. The lacrimal passages are very delicate and a coarsely handled probe may turn a temporary obstruction into a permanent one.

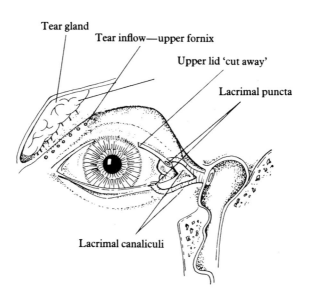

Tear gland

Tear inflow—upper fornix

Upper lid 'cut away'

Lacrimal puncta

Lacrimal canaliculi

Fig. 8.1   The lacrimal apparatus, part of the external quadruple alliance, has much in common with the ureters, the bladder and the urethra. Poorly positioned puncta are a commoner cause of a watering eye than is a blocked nasolacrimal duct. A dry eye is more common than a watering eye.

Adults

A chronic nasal catarrh in our temperate climate may have something to do with the equally common blockage of the nasolacrimal duct.

If surgery be deemed necessary, it involves cracking a hole in the bone between the lacrimal fossa and the nasal cavity. A union is then effected between the lacrimal sac and the nasal mucosa. The operation – a dacryocystorrhinostomy – is not always undertaken with great hope of success because fistulae tend to remain only when unwanted.

It is as well to ask patients if their symptoms are bad enough to make them want such an operation. Indeed a description of the surgical manoeuvring may well be all that is needed.

Simple measures must precede surgery. Topical astringents like zinc sulphate to the eye, together with decongestants to the nose, can sometimes constrict the duct mucosa at both ends. Prolonged application in the nose ends up doing the reverse.

Zinc sulphate is prescribed most commonly in association with adrenaline. Of late, this combination has fallen under suspicion for fear that it might provoke acute angle closure. It can only do so if the anterior chamber is shallow. It seems harsh to deny an eye with a deep anterior chamber the benefits of a useful medication when it is so easy to identify an eye at risk.

Lacrimal sac abscess

The great reservoir is the lacrimal sac, where stagnant tears may explode into a lacrimal abscess – unmistakable as an angry red swelling between the nose and the medial canthus. Pressure on the tear sac – if tolerated – may produce pus at the lacrimal puncta.

Treatment begins with systemic antibiotics as a short term measure.

The long term surgical cure is dacryocystorrhinostomy, which may not appear so repellent an alternative to a lacrimal sac abscess.

Trauma

Rupture of the canaliculus in the lower lid used to be a common windscreen injury before seat belts were enforced by law.

Surgical attempts to reunite the torn ends used to involve arranging them around a silicone tube which was then passed through the upper canaliculus.

The result was often not only obstruction in the lower canaliculus but damage to the upper one as well. Since the upper one has now to do all the work, it is best left alone.

It must not be assumed therefore that all watering is due to blockage along the nasolacrimal duct. If surgery is not contemplated, and there is no evidence of lacrimal sac infection then there is nothing to be gained by invading the ducts with a coarse and possibly infected probe.

If patients did not start off with a lacrimal sac infection, it is not inconceivable that they could end up with it. Simple drops to the eye and nostril are the first move. Threat of surgery is the second, and an actual operation may well be the start of a series.

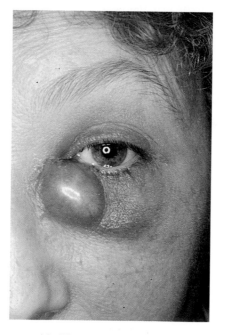

Fig. 8.2   Acute dacryocystitis. Watering is not the most pressing complaint but in time it may become so.

SUMMARY

The basal tear flow keeps the external eye moist.
  The response flow is provoked by irritation.
  Eyes water without an obvious cause when:

1. a deficient basic secretion produces irritation
2. the lids do not contact the globe (ectropion) it need not be gross
3. some malfunction blocks the nasolacrimal duct; this is less common than ectropion.

  Canalicular damage from injury is self evident.

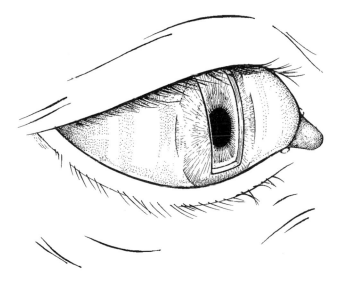

Fig. 8.3 The lid margin in contact with the globe is a vital element in the external quadruple alliance and it must contact the globe snugly to be a successful member of the Imperial Guard for the cornea.

9. Fundal appearances

The dominant feature of the inner eye as seen with the ophthalmoscope is the red reflex. The final degree of redness is a compromise between:

1. the scleral white trying to be seen through
2. the vascular choroid, itself masked by
3. the pigment retina, the density of which will be affected by race, the size of the eye and defects such as albinism
4. the neuro-retina is transparent face on and visible only in profile when detached.

Looking at the fundus is the eighth sign and we should only pick up the ophthalmoscope when we have decided from our evaluation of the seven signs what we are going to see inside the eye.

The direct ophthalmoscope is not an easy instrument to use. It is affected by extremes of refractive error such as aphakia or myopia. It produces a magnified view of the fundus and the price paid for such magnification we see only a small area of the fundus at a time. To use the analogy of microscopy we are going straight to high magnification without first sensing the relationship of adjacent structures through low magnification.

Using the direct ophthalmoscope, we can expect to see the posterior pole only, and for all practical purposes this consists of:

1. the disc
2. vessels in relation to the disc
3. the macula.

Opacities in the cornea, the lens and the vitreous, the wholly baffling reluctance to dilate the pupil and the optical frailties of the direct ophthalmoscope all combine to make fundoscopy an art prized by those who master it and dismissed with some envy by those who do not. There has never been a shortage of those in the middle who settle for the impression of mastery.

This wholly understandable vanity was acknowledged by a well known Edinburgh physician who, pin-striped and elegant, would drape himself around his patient before a gallery of admiring students. When he finally uncurled himself he would announce, 'It doesn't matter what you see, provided you do it with style.'

COMMON FUNDAL APPEARANCES

Senile macular degeneration

Dysfunction in the macular area of one form or another is one of the main causes of visual handicap. It comes in a variety of guises, usually in the over sixties. For many as yet unexplained reasons, the macular retina begins to disintegrate.

Considering its complexity, the wonder is that it does not do so earlier in life. Whichever of its layers primarily gives way, the end result is one or a blend of four things:

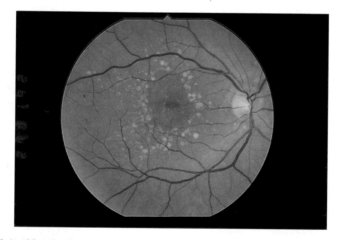

Fig. 9.1   Macular degeneration. Disturbance in the macular area takes the form of either: 1) atrophy – allowing the sclera to shine through; 2) pigmentary disturbance – masking the underlying choroid; or 3) exudation – also masking the underlying choroid. The colloid bodies seen here can be thought of as exudate, although in fact they lie deep to the retina on *Bruch's* membrane. If the visual field is full, as implied by the normal optic nerve head, then the eye is by no means blind.

1. macular atrophy – exposing the white sclera
2. hard exudates masking the choroid and the white sclera
3. abnormal pigmentation masking both choroid and sclera
4. frank haemorrhage masking everything.

The essential question to be decided is whether the degeneration is wet or dry. If dry, it is therefore already atrophic. If wet, on the other hand, it may have become so from an area of focal leakage. Such leakage can be coagulated from time to time by a laser which of course destroys the point of coagulation in order to save the rest.

In the main, however, these degenerations progress mercilessly to total loss of central vision.

The condition is common and those who suffer it must not suffer also the fear that they are going to lose the rest of their vision. It must be assured that blindness will not follow.

We can assure ourselves of this by confirming the absence of glaucoma the process. This of course is common in the age group that suffers macular degeneration. In most cases, visual field loss due to an elevated intraocular pressure can be treated, preserving the patient's capacity to navigate and our reputation for having assured them that they always would be able to do so.

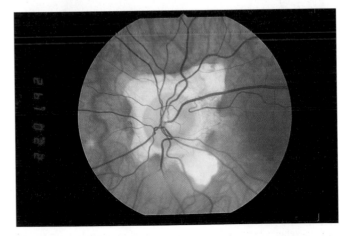

Fig. 9.2 Myopic atrophy. The myopic eye is a large eye, leaving thin areas of choroid and pigment retina through which the white sclera dominates.

Myopia

The short-sighted eye is a big eye. Its layers might be thought to be thinner than standard and occasionally they crack. A crack at the macula is more common in a young myope than in a normally-sighted person of the same age.

Haemorrhage from the choroid may seep through that crack into the neuro-retina, particularly in the macular area, producing a juvenile and myopic version of disciform macular degeneration.

Benign equatorial degeneration

In older age groups a fine-spun interlacing pattern of mottled pigmentation encircles the globe around the equator. The range of the direct ophthalmoscope may extend to include this if the pupil is dilated. Its major significance is the danger that casual observation might lead to a mistaken diagnosis of retinitis pigmentosa.

Retinitis pigmentosa

There is no more emotive condition. Beginning between the ages of 6 and 12, and more common in men than women, this bilateral

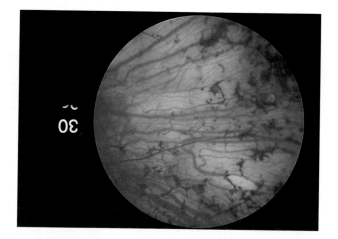

Fig. 9.3   Retinitis pigmentosa – the most celebrated of the retinal degenerations. It has no fixed genetic basis and has been described in virtually every syndrome. It is characterised by night blindness, visual field constriction and a scatter of pigment over the posterior retina in the form of bone corpuscles.

inherited malady leads to total destruction of peripheral retinal function.

A scatter of pigment clumps in the shape of bone corpuscles, recalled from early days with the microscope, creeps around the posterior pole of the retina just behind the equator. As the retina atrophies, so does the ability to see in the dark, with the onset of night blindness.

Then follows a progressive constriction of the visual field until in the fifties only a few degrees of central vision remain.

Tunnel vision is an apt name and we can reproduce the sensation of these awful restrictions by looking down a long narrow tube. Such field constriction is perhaps more common in chronic simple glaucoma simply because chronic simple glaucoma is more common.

Retinitis pigmentosa has prompted much so far fruitless research and many expensive and trumpery remedies. Despite the impressive manipulation of polysyllabic chemicals in remote and picturesque clinics, there is no convincing evidence that any of them does more than introduce yet another alien poison to the system, whilst siphoning off large sums of money into remote bank accounts.

Albinism

The retinal pigment layer plays a vital function in the metabolism of visual pigments as well as absorbing excess light. It is recognized by the classic bleach-white skin and hair of the albino, and the red reflex which can be seen not only through the pupil but through the atrophic iris as well.

Such eyes do not see well, not only because of absent metabolites, but also because the existing retina is overwhelmed by the light presented.

There are other familial progressive and unfortunately untreatable chorioretinal degenerations – whether called choroideremia or gyrate atrophy – all result in night blindness and tunnel vision. Whether this is due to choroidal atrophy or retinal atrophy or both is of little practical comfort to the patient, who just doesn't see well and as the years go by will see even less.

Choroiditis (chorioretinitis)

Arising occasionally in the wake of other diseases, choroiditis is frequently an inflammation in its own right, often without any known cause. Traditional marks of inflammation collect in a patch in the posterior pole, resulting in exudation of inflammatory fluids into the vitreal cavity. The patient may be aware of floaters and possibly blunting of central vision, but little else.

The seven signs will perhaps confirm the visual symptoms, but need not be very remarkable otherwise.

The diagnosis is made from the history, and when floaters are seen through the dilated pupil against the red reflex. A fluffy, white patch may be seen when the retina comes into focus. As with any inflammation, the episode may go on to form a scar. Destruction of more delicate tissues, like the choroid, the pigment and the neuro-retina, allows the sclera to dominate. White is therefore the first element of the scar.

Because there has been an active battle, the one layer that is capable of proliferation will proliferate. Pigment will therefore be seen and, because the end-result of any battle is confusion, such

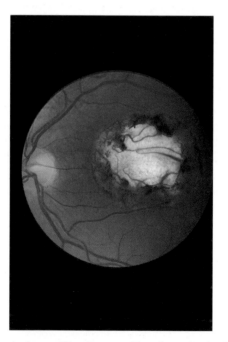

Fig. 9.4   Chorioretinal scar. All such scars, although varying in size and location, essentially look the same. Inflammation destroys the choroid and the two retinae, allowing the white sclera to shine through choroidal remnants. Fragments of pigment are scattered about by the only layer capable of proliferation.

pigment will be scattered irregularly over the white sclera. Pigment clumps and borders are therefore the second component of a chorioretinal scar.

Not everything in the area is totally destroyed and red choroidal remnants join the pigment.

The final appearance therefore will be that of white sclera visible through a broken lacework of chorioretinal remnants – whorls and smudges of black pigment and fibrous tissue in a circumscribed patch surrounded by a normal red reflex.

It is perfectly possible to fill out several chapters on the subject of these scars, but it would also be pointless because, whatever their cause, they are all the same.

They may be different positions and with different distribution – infection with *Toxoplasma* or *Toxocara*, in solitary circumscribed patches that may be of no consequence unless they happen to be on the macula. Fluffy clouds blur their edges when they are preparing to erupt again.

Laser scars are distributed in a regular pattern in a patient who should manage to tell us what has happened.

Cryopexy scars following retinal surgery, eclipse burns and the peppered distribution of syphilitic chorioretinitis that slip from one edition to the next, but somehow never manage to slip into a clinic – they all show the common features of a white sclera dominating through a broken choroid, with pigment clumps to indicate a past struggle.

If chorioretinitis is induced as a result of treatment, then there is no need to treat it. If it is induced by infection, then that is another matter. Systemic corticosteroids in high doses can limit the damage, but they can also produce damage in their own right. If the macula is not directly threatened, there is much to be said for allowing even infective chorioretinitis to follow its own course.

Choroidal melanoma

This is the most common intraocular malignancy – occurring in one eye usually after the age of 50. Because early symptoms are so vague, it usually attracts attention when it is too big to submit to local removal. Ignored, it can fill the cavity of the eye, blocking the drainage angle and causing acute secondary glaucoma. Most often it is picked up as an incidental finding, or when the symptoms of creeping retinal detachment can no longer be ignored.

Metastases spread via the bloodstream, most often, if the favoured description is correct, to the liver.

The tumour is seen with the ophthalmoscope as a solid mottled lump, frequently associated with an adjacent fluid retinal detachment, carried by gravity into the lower part of the eye.

Should the mass be too large for local excision, then the current management is removal of the eye. However, this is a moot point. Diagnosis of these lesions is sometimes extremely difficult and a postoperative discovery that it was actually benign is not always a consolation to the patient, who may have parted with a symptomless eye.

Surgery itself is thought to give rise to a sudden impetus of blood-borne spread, and the old adage 'beware of the one-eyed man with the large liver' must raise a question mark over the wisdom of making him one-eyed in the first place.

Recent progress allowing the excision of tumours has opened the pleasing possibility of preserving vision in eyes that were formerly enucleated.

But against this must be placed the danger of shortening life by disturbing a sleeping tiger that might have continued to slumber.

Some studies suggest that patients with small malignant tumours have the same life expectancy as have a control group equivalent in everything except for the tumour. A disturbing

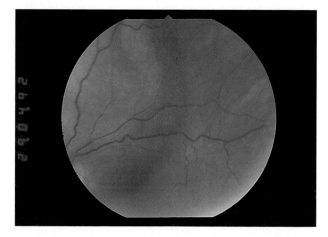

Fig. 9.5   Melanoma – a large, grey-black choroidal tumour displacing the pigment retina and the neuro-retina towards the vitreal cavity. Sometimes associated with fluid separation of the neuro-retina from the pigment retina.

thought that arises from that, however, is that all big tumours must have been small at one time.

Comparison of serial photographs over several months is perhaps the best compromise between instant enucleation and optimistic discharge from hospital care.

Of course we must always exclude the possibility that what is taken for primary tumour may in fact be secondary to a mass elsewhere.

Haemorrhage

In a recent collection of 'instant syndromes for busy residents', there featured a colour plate of a retinal haemorrhage – shaped like a sea-anemone and with the legend 'lymphatic leukaemia'.

The most dangerous feature of the plate was not the lymphatic leukaemia, but the inference that every other leukaemia might have a unique counterpart somewhere on the sea-bed.

The retinal haemorrhage of course was diagnostic of blood and nothing more.

Bleeding within the eye occurs, as does bleeding anywhere, for one of three reasons:

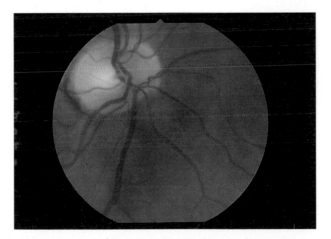

Fig. 9.6 Choroidal naevus. These freckles are frequently seen in the normal fundus, where fears about normality are raised. Their uniform blackness and sharp edges mark them as benign now and benign indefinitely. A malignant melanoma in its early stages adds a muddy greyness to the absence of all the other above qualities.

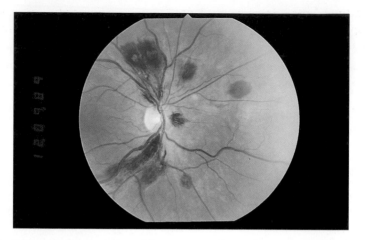

Fig. 9.7 Retinal haemorrhage. The appearance is not diagnostic of anything other than haemorrhage. It may follow trauma or one of the bleeding disorders or spontaneous dissolution of the macular layers. The central red haemorrhage is related to the neuro-retina. The darker grey lies beneath the pigment retina.

1. disturbance of the blood
2. disturbance of the blood vessels
3. disturbance of the blood pressure.

Any leukaemia can certainly disturb the blood, but so can warfarin or simple anaemia.

Disease can reduce the integrity of blood vessels; hypoxia can create new vessels; a retinal tear or a sudden reduction in intraocular pressure can produce haemorrhage from normal vessels.

Fluctuations in blood pressure are just another reminder that ophthalmic investigations may start in the eye, but can lead anywhere.

Phakomatoses

These are included for completeness. A rare collection of lumps scattered throughout the body as well as the eye, and hovering uneasily between the title of genuine tumour and embryonic remnants, their names read like characters from a Lehar operetta: Von Recklinghausen, Von Hippel–Lindau, Bourneville and Sturge-Weber.

Café au lait spots, skin tumours, intracranial gliomata, angiomatous malformations, sebaceous adenomata and so on will produce local damage and disorder wherever they alight. Unpredictable to some degree, fortunately they are as rare as they are untreatable.

SUMMARY

The ophthalmoscope should be picked up only when we have decided from the seven signs what the eighth sign is going to tell us.

Our attempts can be foiled by:

1. opacities in the cornea, lens, vitreous
2. severe myopia
3. aphakia
4. poor co-operation.

The red reflex is a compromise appearance between:

1. scleral white
2. the choroidal red
3. the pigment black
4. the transparent-when-flat neuro-retina.

10. Retinal detachment

The inside of the eye is rather like a brandy goblet lined with fine cellophane. This cellophane is attached at the rim and at the stem and is potentially separable everywhere else. The rim corresponds to the ora serrata – the anterior limit of the functioning retina and deep to a line connecting the insertions of the four rectus muscles.

Anterior to that line the two layers unite and fuse into a composite epithelium which lines the inner surface of the ciliary body. This epithelium secreting aqueous is the heart of the eye.

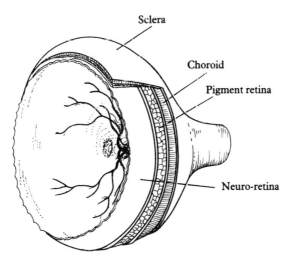

Fig. 10.1 The ocular brandy goblet. The rim is of smaller diameter than the equator. There are four main ocular layers.

PATHOLOGICAL BASIS

A retinal detachment occurs when the inner cellophane layer (the neuro-retina) separates from the outer layer (the pigment retina). It may do so for three reasons of which the first is the most common:

1. spontaneous separation with liquified vitreous passing through a hole in the neuro-retina into the potential space
2. the neuro-retina may be pulled into the vitreal cavity by traction
3. the neuro-retina may be pushed off by some space-occupying lesion or by choroidal effusion on its deep surface.

The vitreous body, transparent like a half-set jelly, is also attached to the retina at the same two points, namely the ora serrata (the rim) and the optic nerve head (the stem). It is more loosely attached to a third point – the macula. The healthy vitreous – viscous and thick – acts as a shock-absorber whilst keeping the retina in place. However, passing years can reduce its viscosity, a process exaggerated by inflammation, injury or extreme myopia and given the name of syneresis.

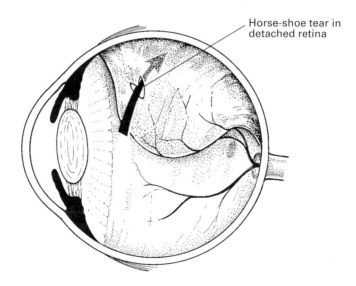

Horse-shoe tear in detached retina

Fig. 10.2 Retinal detachment is actually separation of the neuro-retina from the pigment retina by degenerate vitreous, which passes through a break into the potential space between them.

Liquifaction of the vitreous on its own cannot bring about a retinal detachment. It can, however, in association with another flaw.

If for reasons to be explained later, a break forms in the neural layer, then this syneretic vitreous is now fluid enough to pass through into the potential space, producing that separation of the two layers that we call retinal detachment.

The essential point is that neither a liquid vitreous alone nor a retinal break alone can bring about this separation. They have to act in concert.

Abnormal adhesion between the vitreous and the retina facilitates the formation of a retinal break. Continued traction by the vitreous on such an adhesion stimulates the retina into the only response of which it is capable – continued flashes of light. This light flashing is not a symptom of a detaching retina but a tearing retina.

Once the break is complete, the light flashing stops. Rupture of a vessel at this point may fill the vitreal cavity with blood, described by the patient as a sudden shower of floaters – like a swarm of bees.

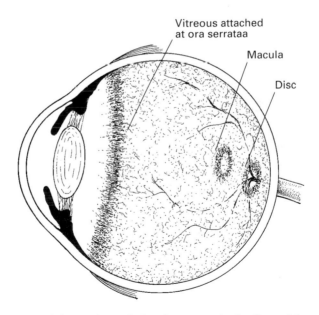

Fig. 10.3   Normal vitreous is attached to the ora serrata, the disc and the macula. Uncontrolled loss of vitreous drags on all three. The commonest cause of uncontrolled vitreal loss is a cataract extraction that goes wrong.

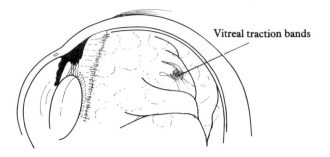

Fig. 10.4 Abnormal vitreal adhesions drag light flashes out of the retina until they eventually drag a piece of retina out of the retina, when the light flashes give way to floaters which in turn give way to black shadow as the retina detaches.

The lifting neuro-retina produces a black shadow or curtain dominant in one section of the visual field.

If sudden, symptoms are dramatic. If less sudden, they could well be ignored until the separating retina lifts the macula and sets the alarm bells ringing months or even years after the process began.

Separation of the neuro-retina from the pigment layer is not just an immediate visual disaster. There is a potential for even greater disaster in the long term. The neuro-retina depends on the pigment layer for sustenance which is withheld when the layers are separated. If the detachment goes on long enough untreated, the retina will starve to death, becoming in the process so fibrotic that mechanical replacement would be impossible even if enough functioning retina remained to justify the attempt.

No matter what the underlying cause, all retinal detachments, unless a vitreal haemorrhage has obscured the fundal view, are characterized by a grey reflex rippling in place of the normal red. The retina, transparent face on, becomes opaque and in profile it obscures the underlying choroidal red glow and the underlying choroidal detail.

Retinal breaks develop in four main ways, with a fifth rarity:

Myopic

The myopic eye is almost too big for its own contents. It is rather like a large slice of toast partially covered with a small pat of butter. It is these partially covered areas that are dangerous. They

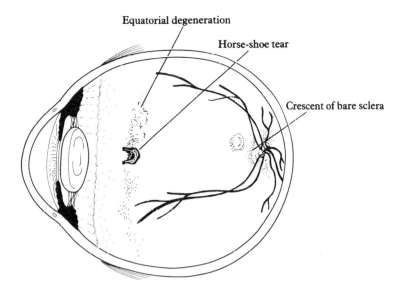

Equatorial degeneration

Horse-shoe tear

Crescent of bare sclera

Fig. 10.5 The short-sighted eye is too big for its own good. Distance vision focuses short of the retina. Its layers are thin and almost absent in areas like a small pat of butter trying to cover a large slice of toast. A crack at the macula can ruin central vision. A crack at the equator can cause a detached retina.

are thinner than standard retina and the whole myopic retina is thinner anyway. In addition, abnormal vitreous adheres to the attenuated areas and in time tugs on the retina, producing flashing lights which give way to floaters as the retina itself gives way into a retinal break or tear.

Naturally such eyes and such patients are vulnerable to trauma, sudden head movements and general agitation than are those with normal eyes. As a fair proportion of virtuoso musicians are also short-sighted it is perhaps a wonder that more of them are not carried from the keyboard with sparks flying in the wake of a savage cadenza.

Congenital

The greatest activity demanded by the developing retina is in the lower temporal region and it is not surprising that development is not always complete. These cracks behind and parallel to the ora serrata exist as a fault and not as a happening. There is therefore neither traction nor light flashing. The vitreous being healthy and

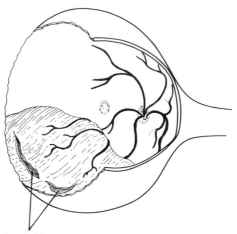

Break just behind ora serrata

Fig. 10.6 The delayed result of either a congenital defect or trauma. Gravity and a thick vitreous delay the onset of the detachment. The ocular 'brandy goblet' is very evident in this illustration.

equally innocent is not sufficiently liquified to pass through the break which is thus totally without symptoms.

In due course the vitreous does liquify and may quietly pass into the subretinal space. The liquid elevation produces irritation which in turn produces inflammation which in turn produces an inflammatory scar – a thin black line which opposes the advancing detachment. These defensive lines (retinal tide marks) curve like a line of battle with the centre nearest the optic nerve head and the flanks curving towards the ora serrata.

In time the detachment advances again and another defensive line forms. Several lines may form without the patient's knowing until the final advance into the macular region at which point the distress signals sound for urgent loss of vision – demonstrating yet again that central vision is the only element of vision that people know they have.

Traumatic

Injury to an eye can be blunt or lacerating.

Shock waves from a blow produce contre-coup holes in the line of the injury. They can also produce a break near the ora serrata.

They are more likely to rip the actual ora serrata itself from its moorings. Thereafter, if left to its own devices the eye may settle and develop a detachment not very different from that produced by a congenital crack.

It must always be remembered, however, that eyes that have suffered such a blow can also suffer other affects from the same blow, namely dislocation of the lens and scarring of the trabecular meshwork. In youth this destruction of the drainage meshwork may not be terribly obvious because a young eye has great reserves of pressure control. However, as age erodes these reserves, meshwork damage, perhaps long forgotten, will be revealed by an asymptomatic rise in intraocular pressure, detected in time only if someone looks for it.

Lacerating trauma involves tearing of the retina with a sharp edge and precise location of such a tear will depend on where the edge falls. It will generally occur in two ways – either from a foreign body entering the cavity of the eye, usually through the front, or by some agency such as a piece of windscreen glass slicing the globe directly.

Aphakic

The advent of extracapsular extraction has reduced the incidence of detachment following cataract surgery enormously. When a cataract is removed by the intracapsular technique, the vitreal cavity loses its anterior wall. The vitreous moves forwards to occupy the space once occupied by the lens, dragging holes in the peripheral attachment of the retina often years after the original cataract extraction.

Macular

For completeness we ought to remember that a fifth and much rarer retinal hole may develop in the macula itself – usually a consequence of myopia but possibly following trauma and indeed of its own accord without any demonstrable underlying disease.

CLINICAL FEATURES

The larger the break and the further it is above the horizontal meridian, the more thin the vitreous, the more dramatic will be the symptoms.

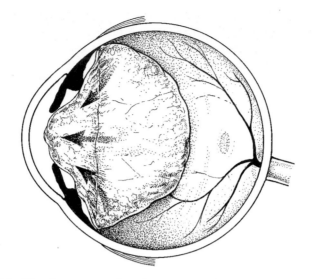

Fig. 10.7   The vitreous moves into the space vacated by the lens and drags on the retina at the ora. The ensuing retinal break cannot be seen with the direct ophthalmoscope.

Conversely inferior breaks in otherwise healthy eyes will be asymptomatic until the macula is affected.

Most people are not aware of creeping field loss but will report a sudden shadow.

1. & 2. *Central vision – distance* and *near*: may be normal, slightly blunted or grossly affected
3. *Field vision*: will confirm a defect where a shadow has been reported.
5. *Pupil*: a sluggish reflex to light indicates a poorly functioning retina.
7. *Intraocular pressure*: may be significantly low compared with that of the other side.

Fundus: a view through the dilated pupil will reveal a grey reflex rippling over a lost choroidal pattern in the area corresponding to the reported shadow and to the defect picked up in the visual field.

MANAGEMENT

A recent detachment is always an ocular emergency, particularly if the macula is intact.

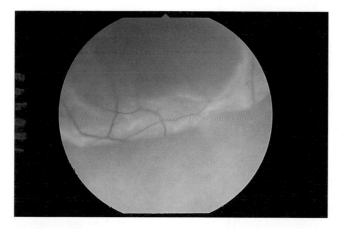

Fig. 10.8   Retinal detachment. Separation of the retina becomes obvious when the choroidal pattern is increasingly lost behind deepening subretinal fluid.

Within the framework of treatment principles there is no medical treatment for a retinal detachment caused by a hole in the retina.

But surgical treatment really means surgery and not 'laser welding'. Although the popular scientific press frequently would suggest the contrary, with a wealth of descriptive detail, it is impossible to treat a detachment of the retina with a laser.

Short term management

Bed rest in an appropriate position will often allow gravity to protect the macula from collecting subretinal fluid.

Long term management

The first step to successful retinal surgery is to find the causative break – a manoeuvre best achieved with the indirect ophthalmoscope. There is nothing like a retinal detachment to expose the optical weaknesses of anything else.

The second aim is to seal that tear against further passage of liquified vitreous. The seal is induced by inflammatory scar. The inflammation is produced by freezing. The freezing spots can be aimed with great precision from outside the sclera delivering a low temperature through all the ocular layers to the pigment retina and to the neuro-retina around the retinal break.

Sealing the tear alone may not be enough because the traction which produced the original break may still be under tension and could well pull the break open again.

There are a variety of ways to prevent this but the common factor is a segment of silicone rubber or silicone-based sponge which is stitched under tension to the sclera to raise a mound directly beneath the retinal break in all the layers together and hopefully preventing them from separating.

In addition the volume of the eye can be generally reduced by encircling the equator with a band of silicone rubber, stitched to the sclera, which can be also used to modify the position of the local segment.

These explants very occasionally find their way to the surface of the conjunctiva as foreign bodies and if they are a source of irri-

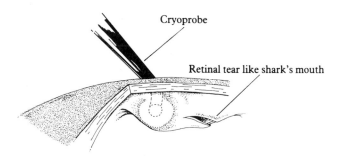

Fig. 10.9   The tear is sealed with an inflammatory scar. The inflammation can be produced by 'frostbite'. If the retina is detached, such inflammation cannot be produced with the laser. Recent advances suggest that the once abandoned diathermy may be making a comeback.

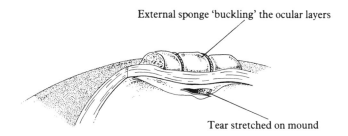

Fig. 10.10   A silicone sponge, stitched to the outside of the eye, raises a mound inside on which a tear is held until inflammation seals it with a scar.

tation can be removed with much greater simplicity than their appearance might suggest.

If the previous manoeuvres cannot seal the tear to the liking of the surgeon, then air or a mixture of air and a gas like sulphur hexafluoride (SF6), which is less quickly absorbed, can be injected into the vitreal cavity to float the retina upwards and to seal the break from within by surface tension.

The fluid collected under the retina can be left to absorb spontaneously or if its presence impedes surgery it can be released by a separate incision through the sclera, choroid and pigment retina.

There is no single type of retinal operation and surgeons have preferences which they cannot always explain to others. In essence, all surgery is a series of manoeuvres which can be deployed in sequence as the behaviour of the eye demands. The limiting factor is the patency of the central retinal artery and any technique has to make space within the eye to allow the manoeuvre to be carried out, be it air injection or scleral buckling or both, without obstructing the flow of blood through the central retinal artery.

Patients are sometimes positioned after surgery to allow the tear to float on the summit of an air bubble which always rises to the highest point of the eye. Otherwise, the treatment is that of

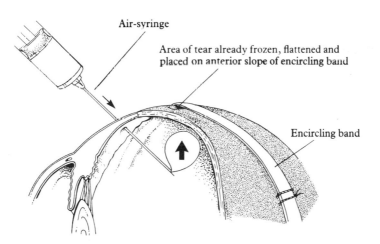

Fig. 10.11   Air in the vitreous can close the edges of the tear by surface tension. The technique is of long pedigree and with good reason – air is effective, cheap and non-toxic.

any other iritis, whatever the cause – topical mydriatics and topical corticosteroids.

The eye should settle within a few days and the patient should be back to normal within a month. There is a long tradition of misery as an essential part of management with appalling tales of debilitating bed rest prolonged and made more miserable still by padding both eyes and a diet of gruel. These contribute nothing to the well-being of the patient or the retina and belong to the pages of a book which should now be firmly closed.

Whatever the technique chosen, the success rate should be of the order of 95%. The 5% fail essentially because of retinal shrinkage for reasons that have never been wholly explained.

Vitrectomy

Described in the section on advanced proliferative diabetic retinopathy, this manoeuvre has extended the surgical repertoire against detachments that used to be considered shrunken beyond all conventional methods.

The prospects are exciting and include total removal of the vitreous, replacement of the vitreous with silicone oil to force the retina into place, section of traction bands throughout the vitreal cavity, peeling of membranes from the surface of the retina and generally doing things that were considered unimaginable in the not very distant past.

It must be remembered that all such stratagems are perforating injuries in their own right and as such can be a potential, though rare, cause of sympathetic ophthalmitis – itself a disease of some rarity.

RETINAL DETACHMENT NOT DUE TO A RETINAL BREAK

The fibrous bands and puckering membranes of diabetic retinopathy may drag the retina into the vitreal cavity rather like an inverted umbrella.

Traction within the vitreal cavity

Trauma, particularly that involving haemorrhage into the vitreous, not infrequently produces the same picture.

Displacement of the retina from without

Choroidal tumour

Primary or secondary malignant masses in the choroid stimulate fluid collection beneath the adjacent retina. The primary if small enough can be removed without the loss of the eye. If small enough it may also be missed altogether as a cause of the detachment.

The treatment of secondary masses is of course the treatment of the primary.

Subretinal effusion

Inflammation of the sclera or of the choroid may fill the potential space between the two retinae with inflammatory fluid. The management of such effusions is not always very satisfactory but in principle must involve elimination of the underlying cause if that is possible. Such a cause might be inflammation of the sclera (scleritis), a process usually idiopathic but possibly rheumatic in origin, rare for either reason and usually resistant to systemic corticosteroids. Disappearance of the subretinal fluid would follow suppression of the inflammation.

SUMMARY

There are two retinal layers – neural and pigment. The pigment layer adheres to the choroid. The neuro-retina adheres only at the ora serrata and the optic nerve head. A potential space exists between them.

Detachment of the retina is most commonly caused by a retinal break, which may be:

1. *myopic* – eye bigger than standard
2. *congenital* – developmental crack in the peripheral retina
3. *traumatic* (blunt or lacerating) – complicated by vitreal haemorrhage producing traction
4. *aphakic* – vitreal shift at ora serrata. Incidence reduced by extra-capsular extraction
5. *macular hole.*

Danger: blindness from retinal starvation and shrinkage.

Management:

1. Find the break.
2. Inflame the pigment retina around break with freezing.
3. Hold the break against inflamed area long enough to produce a watertight scar.

Less common causes of detached retina are:

1. traction in the vitreal cavity
2. displacement from the outer layers.

It is an established part of ophthalmic folklore and the quasi-scientific press that the answer to a detached retina is a laser, which cures the problem in a flash, with no need for anaesthesia, surgery or a hospital bed. This is, alas, nonsense.

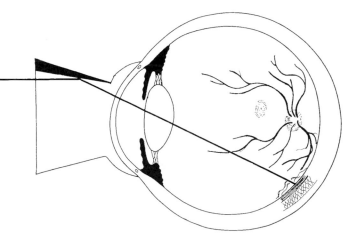

Fig. 10.12 The laser is reflected off a mirror through a contact lens to the pigment retina, where it is absorbed, then released as heat to coagulate anything in contact. If the retina is detached, the laser can have no place in its treatment.

Laser is a light which, when picked up by the pigment retina, is turned into heat which then coagulates anything lying in contact. 'Lying in contact' is the rub. A detached retina is not in contact and therefore not only escapes the coagulating beam but also prevents that beam from reading the pigment retina in the first place.

11. Cataract

The natural lens has one fundamental answer to insult: it becomes opaque. Different degree of insult cause different degrees of opacity but whatever their degree we call them all cataract. Here we have yet another example of the single response – another terminus at which lines from every direction arrive. All the tissues of the eye are susceptible to the same conditions that plague the rest of the body. From the common list of causation, we can develop a host of possible reasons why the lens should become opaque.

Congenital

Maternal infection with, say German measles (rubella) during the first trimester of pregnancy will catch the lens nucleus, whilst infection later will be reflected in opacities further into the cortex.

Hereditary

There may be a familial tendency to cataract formation at any age – though more worthy of comment in the young.

Traumatic

Contusion injuries and penetrating injuries, of which intraocular surgery for glaucoma is an example, may disturb the fluids around the lens sufficiently to disturb the lens itself. Actual rupture of the lens capsule with windscreen glass or a metallic foreign body rapidly produces a total cataract.

Inflammatory

Iritis grumbling over a long period reduces the quality of aqueous around the lens. Opacities therefore begin in the lens cortex nearest to the poisoned aqueous.

Neoplastic

No tumour arises directly from the lens but should one grow, as it occasionally does, from the ciliary body it could be near enough the lens capsule to threaten its integrity, with the usual single response.

Metabolic

The fluctuating sugar levels of diabetes give rise to fluctuating fluid balance across the lens capsule. The result at first is fluctuating change in the spectacle requirements of the eye, until the inevitable cataract makes spectacle changes pointless.

Radiational

Most forms of ionizing radiation must be regarded as potentially dangerous but it has yet to be proved that the concealed emanations from television screens or visual display units can seriously affect the eye.

The wave lengths in the infra-red are another matter and some people face them in their daily occupation. A classic victim is the glass blower, paying a long-term price for the transient pleasure of gazing in admiration at his molten creations.

Fat dogs, whose only exercise is to blink their eyelids from time to time before a grate ablaze with logs, do not require crystal-clear vision to lumber from one side of the hearth to the other.

Toxic

Corticosteroids in high doses over long periods generally have some unpleasant side effects. Cataract is one such effect but we may have to accept that as the reasonable price of treating something worse.

Degenerative

The lens shares a common origin with skin and hair. As time passes, the skin becomes less elastic and the hair white. The lens always does the first and may also do the second.

Other degenerations exist. In progressive myopia there is an overall decline in ocular function, and cataract at an early age is but one of them.

PATHOLOGY

Various happenings take place within the lens substance. Over-hydration to begin with gives way to dehydration. Degradation of the lens proteins and alteration in the electrolytes have also been recorded, but in too disconnected a fashion to be turned into a therapeutic arrest or actual reversal.

Needless to say this has not dissuaded mountebanks from peddling a variety of nostrums guaranteed to restore clarity – some based on fancy, others on alleged research. It is a kindness to name none of them.

As the water content of the lens rises, so does its refractive power, thus shortening the focusing distance within the eye. Such eyes lose vision in the distance, but gain for near – a startling and welcome development to people who have long struggled with reading glasses.

It would not be human to miss the chance of turning this frailty into an attribute. Discarding reading glasses becomes the miracle of the second sight, which unfortunately does not give way to a third sight until the offending cataract is removed.

The primary effect of cataract is to diminish central vision for near and distance. The field of vision generally suffers later. Rarely, the lens may become swollen like a ripe plum, and indeed may burst within the eye, releasing toxic material into the anterior chamber, where it may do all the things that a severe acute iritis might do.

SYMPTOMS

The responses of patients to developing cataract are variations on the theme of visual disturbance. There is an overall blunting of

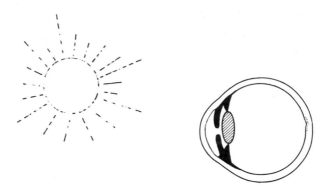

Fig. 11.1 Vision worse in the sunlight means some opacity exaggerated by a pupil constriction – usually cataract.

vision. Excessive sunlight constricts the pupil, exaggerating the opacity behind it. The altered structure of the lens adds an orange glow to entering light. The word halo is mentioned but it is not the 'rainbow' halo of acute angle closure.

Vision is occasionally split by the cataract, with the resultant complaint of double vision. It is of course genuine double vision but affecting one eye only – a fact that can be proved by covering the other side. Going through the seven signs will reveal the cataract and all we need do is decide if the cataract is sufficient to account for the visual loss.

The seven signs:

1. *Central vision* – distance: diminished.
2. *Central vision* – near: possibly only slightly blunted to begin with.
3. *Field vision*: unaffected.
4. *Cornea*: clear, but this is the age group of the arcus senilis.
5. *Pupil*: a brisk light reflex indicates a healthy retina; a sluggish light reflex might indicate an unhealthy retina but also might indicate a very dense cataract.
6. *Anterior chamber*: normal unless
   a. a grossly swollen cataract has made it shallow
   b. the patient is an incidental candidate for angle closure.
7. *Intraocular pressure*: there is no reason for this to be raised. The patient, however, is generally in the older age group and may well be old enough to have chronic glaucoma as well.

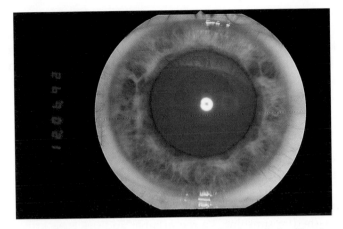

Fig. 11.2   Cataract – best seen against the red reflex through the dilated pupil with an ophthalmoscope held some 20 cm away from the eye.

Patients in the younger age group could have acquired their cataract because of trauma, which in turn may have caused a secondary rise in pressure.

MANAGEMENT

What action, if any, hinges around one single question: is the visual acuity bad enough to justify cataract extraction?

Such an extraction, if successful, is the only way to eliminate this visual impediment: despite the expensive blandishments of some pharmaceutical companies there is no medical way to make the natural lens clear again.

Were it not for the advent of the intraocular lens implant, there would still be a powerful argument for delaying cataract extraction as long as possible.

After a cataract has been removed the eye has to be corrected with a strong convex lens – equal in power to the one extracted.

Such vision is certainly different and possibly unwelcome. It is different because the correcting lens has to sit in a spectacle frame somewhere ahead of the natural position of the natural lens. It may be unwelcome because of magnification. Magnification anywhere increases the image at the expense of the field, which is markedly reduced and sharp-edged with no feathering at its peripheral margins.

The result is a world of magnified images that enter and leave a restricted field without warning. It is for this reason that an aphakic eye (lens removed) cannot make a binocular union with a normal eye using standard glasses. It is also for this reason that strenuous attempts have been made to find an alternative to standard glasses.

Short term (medical)

In the early stages it is possible to improve vision by permanent dilatation of the pupil with, say, atropine drops perhaps three times weekly. Tinting the glasses with sodium yellow allows light to enter, but not to dazzle. It has the quality of making every day seem bathed in sunshine – a remarkable and priceless attribute in a British January.

Long term (surgical)

Extraction is the only effective cure. It does not actually remove the cause because the cause is unknown but it does remove the effects of the cause.

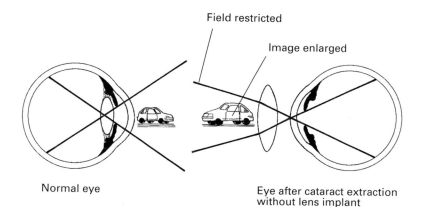

Fig. 11.3   Normal eye – normal image, large field. Aphakic eye – magnified image, small field. It is the horrors of aphakia that led to the development of intraocular lens implantation.

SURGERY

Cataract extraction

The natural lens whether it be clear or opaque is shaped rather like a lentil with the inner structure of a plum. The essential question is how to deliver the plum stone – the nucleus?

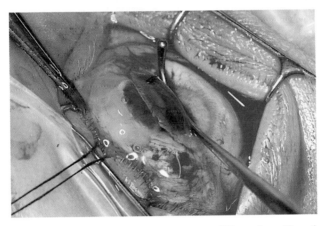

Fig. 11.4 Cataract extraction. The lens is structured like a plum. Here the nucleus and some cortex is expelled. Any remaining cortex can be washed away.

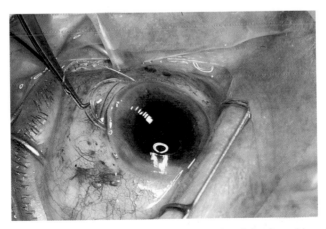

Fig. 11.5 Intraocular lens implantation. A Perspex lens is implanted into the capsular sac, compensating for the optical structure just removed.

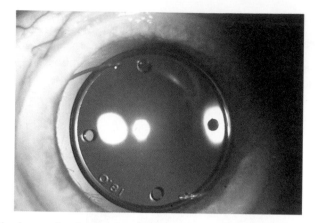

Fig. 11.6 A posterior chamber lens implant in place and seen clearly against the red reflex through the dilated pupil.

Extracapsular extraction

The popular method today is the so-called extracapsular extraction, a refinement of the original operation which for want of such refinement went out of favour before the Second World War.

The aim is to remove everything except the posterior skin of the plum (posterior capsule) which leaves the vitreal cavity, behind the pupil, intact and inviolate.

A hole is cut in the anterior skin (anterior capsule) through which the plum stone (the nucleus) is delivered. Then the plum flesh (cortex) is aspirated.

If a Perspex artificial lens is to replace the lost focus, then it is inserted at this time behind the iris.

None of these manoeuvres can be carried out without cutting a section into the eye at the corneo-scleral limbus. At present, the technique requires an incision of at least 120° and such an incision requires to be stitched afterwards. The operation produces a surgical iritis which behaves like any other iritis and can be managed like any other iritis.

Making up for the lost focus

Aphakic spectacles

Not so long ago the only serious correction was a thick lens placed on a standard spectacle frame. Optical defects were ghastly, producing huge magnification in a small field and indeed it is this very optical horror that gave rise to the popular notion of waiting for a cataract to be ready. What we were in fact waiting for was the vision to be so bad that whatever it was after the operation it could only be better than it was before.

We went to great lengths to delay surgery to the point that convalescents would not think back with nostalgia to the second-rate faculty they so blithely exchanged for the unfulfilled hope of something better.

Contact lens

An optical correction placed on the cornea lies much nearer the position vacated by the natural lens. Unfortunately it lies on the outside of the eye and, whatever it is called, it is still a corneal foreign body.

Such foreign bodies can produce infection, irritation and, since they cover much of the corneal surface, can deprive the corneal epithelium of oxygen.

Lens implant

It is because of the problems experienced by cataract glasses and contact lenses and also because of a restless desire to improve upon nature that the idea of the lens implant took root. It came into flower during the Second World War. Up till that time it was and indeed is widely recognized that retained intraocular foreign bodies – and they were not uncommon between 1939 and 1945 – invariably destroyed the eye by moving within and forming toxic salts with the ocular fluids.

There was, however, one exception – aircraft windscreens. Perspex from these fragments lay within the eye and were chemically inert. Misfortune for the brave men who suffered these injuries turned into good fortune for others in the fullness of time. Nowadays there is a lens to suit all tastes – rigid and flexible, before the iris and behind the iris. Although differing in all these ways they share the common element – Perspex.

The technique naturally adds gratuitous dangers to an operation that is not without its own risks. However, despite its rare potential for complicating something simple into something catastrophic, the surgical question now about these implants has irreversibly changed from why to why not?

Indications for extraction

In the adult

Surgery is justified for two essential reasons:

1. when the cataract is significantly interfering with vision
2. when the cataract has become a danger to the eye.

Visual standards: We should never interfere in the name of treatment, unless we feel that our patient is going to be better off as a result. If patients are seeing sufficiently to move around happily in their own environment, then they are best left alone. What constitutes happy movement will of course differ from person to person. Some people may be unhappy at 6/12 whilst others find the idea of surgery ridiculous even at 6/24.

However the Vehicle Licencing Authorities or, more to the point, the police demand 6/12 or better to make out the details of a number plate at 25 yards. 'That of course is the central visual level only. There is also the field to consider.'

But there is more to driving than seeing the number of a registration plate. It is pointless to achieve the driving standard but not to achieve it quickly enough to respond to the sight of an unexpected vehicle.

If it is decided that a driving licence is not top priority, then many years may pass between not making out a number plate at 25 yards and not making out very much at 25 yards. A good working rule is to make sure that our patients want to see better before we refer them for surgery.

A dangerous lens: The development of a cataract is usually so slow that we may fail to recognize that it has matured to the point of bursting. Occasionally such a lens may become over-ripe, rather like a fat plum when the wasps are going frantic. Such lenses can be recognized from their uniform grey-whiteness when no cortex can be detected with a focusing torch.

Should such a lens burst within the eye, it floods it with foreign protein provoking a severe iritis.

This iritis is not unique because it is produced by the lens. It behaves like any other iritis and each affected part will produce its customary single response. The only difference is that the reactive inflammation will not settle until the offending lens has been removed. Operating in a storm is best avoided but if the inflammation cannot be tamed and the intraocular pressure cannot be reduced, then we still have to remove the lens, since leaving it can only turn the storm into something worse.

A cataract can become a source of danger for less dramatic but no less compelling reasons. By preventing a view into the eye it sometimes makes impossible the effective management of lesions such as retinal tears, retinal detachment or diabetic retinopathy.

By preventing a view out of the eye it can break the binocular lock leading to diverging eyes that may not come together again after the offending lens is removed. Our patient will not be grateful for successful restoration of sight if instead of one vision, there are now two.

In the child

The indications for extraction in a child are very similar to those of an adult except for one addition. Up to the age of 5, macular vision is still not finally established. Any impediment to its establishment must therefore be regarded with suspicion. Congenital cataract or indeed any other sort of cataract which effectively threatens visual development in these early years will have to be removed if we are to avoid deprivation amblyopia.

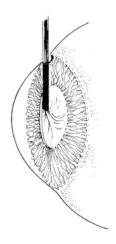

Fig. 11.7 The soft nucleus of youth reduces cataract extraction to simple aspiration.

Naturally some sort of optical correction will have to compensate for the natural lens. In the United States many surgeons would not hesitate to do so with an intraocular lens implant. We are possibly a trifle more conservative in Britain and would at least try first of all to correct the aphakia with a contact lens.

There is, however, another possibility causing much interest all over the world – epikeratophakia. A button of donor cornea with the dioptric equivalent of a lens implant or a contact lens is placed not on the front of the recipient cornea but in the front of it acquiring in time a covering of natural epithelium.

Whatever the possible problems on the outside of the eye, they may outweigh the as yet uncalculated hazards to the inner eye of decades of Perspex implantation.

DISLOCATION OF THE LENS

Spontaneous

Lens dislocation can occur as part of a generalized malfunction of ligament and elastic tissue. The tall, spidery patients described by Marfan and the short stubby ones described by Marchesani both shared defective joints and dislocated lenses.

If the lens stays in the correct plane after it has slipped, then there may be only slight visual distortion.

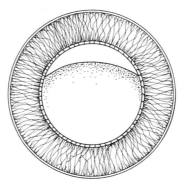

Fig. 11.8   Dislocation of the lens. The optical problem is to decide whether to look around or through the lens. With extreme mobility, such a decision may change from minute to minute. Dislocation into the anterior chamber can have catastrophic effects on the aqueous outflow.

Forward movement can damage the cornea and disturb aqueous dynamics in the anterior chamber.

Backward movement into the vitreal cavity sometimes results in the release of these protein breakdown products responsible for a lens-induced iritis. They are particularly toxic to the eye and, since the lens continues to lie in the posterior cavity, leaking like a damaged oil well, they can in the end of the day destroy the eye altogether.

Traumatic

Blunt trauma, the most common cause, takes us into the world of breaches of the peace and impromptu scuffles so common in hostelries throughout the ages. It also, however, takes us into the old world of the travelling charlatan, the most famous of whom was the Chevalier Taylor. He, amongst others, elevated the posterior dislocation of the lens into an operation which was called 'couching the cataract'. The lens was toppled swiftly either by a flicked thumb nail or by an actual needle plunged through the pupil.

Vision was magically restored long enough for gratitude to translate itself in a more negotiable form. However, before the first hint that things might be going wrong the travellers demonstrated again their talent for rapid movements by decamping with their local reputation possibly irretrievable but their fees already cashed.

Relief from infirmity has almost always been a lucrative pursuit for the travelling quack. The Chevalier was no exception and he travelled far, as he continually had to, in great style.

SUMMARY

The lens is like a flattened transparent plum – stone, flesh and skin being equivalent to nucleus, cortex and capsule.

Any opacity is a cataract. Only the nucleus and the cortex however become opaque. The capsule is always clear.

Extraction is indicated at all ages:

1. for visual reasons
2. because the lens is dangerous

and, in childhood,

3.   to allow the development of central vision.

Extracapsular extraction is the operation of choice today.

The eye is an optical system. Removing the cataract removes a major part of its focusing capacity. Removal alone, without optical correction, can only benefit the extreme myope whose focus, close to the face, is the product of too much focusing power to begin with.

Thick cataract glasses magnify the image and reduce the field.

Contact lenses, nearer the position of the natural lens, reduce that image and widen the field.

Intraocular lens implants, almost in the plane of the natural lens, restore the image and field to their natural size.

12. Glaucoma

The trouble with the word 'glaucoma' is that it staggers beneath the burden of at least six meanings. Since we ophthalmologists tend to slide from one meaning to another without being aware that we have done so, it is not surprising that most other people rarely know when we have and would probably not recognize the difference if they did.

We cannot blame English – a language rich in homonyms – because the confusion is translated into most languages.

When the word glaucoma is used, and it is too firmly embedded in ophthalmic practice to be discarded, it can mean any one of the following:

1. a pathological process
2. any casual rise in intraocular pressure
3. any rise in intraocular pressure for which some agency has been identified
4. the named disease chronic simple glaucoma
5. the named disease acute glaucoma (angle closure)
6. the named disease infantile glaucoma.

To make matters worse the term 'glaucoma' derives from the Greek word for cataract. Literature abounds with descriptions of glaucous eyes, tinged green, and dim from progressing lens opacities. In more recent times, when many eyes ended up both blind and green from as many causes, the term glaucoma was applied to all of them.

Spreading knowledge has now renamed most of them according to their special pathology. But glaucoma, which does not turn the eye green, has retained the term 'glaucoma', whilst the original condition which actually did is now called cataract – alas!

The tussocks of reason leading us out of this swamp are founded in a simple grasp of:

1. the mechanism of pressure control
2. how the mechanism may be disturbed
3. the implications of such disturbance
4. how words other than glaucoma can adequately describe what we are trying to describe.

Normal intraocular pressure

As explained in the first chapter, the aqueous system differs from blood in two distinct ways:

1. aqueous is clear
2. the circulation is not part of a fixed volume system.

Were aqueous as opaque as blood then the eye would survive but not as a transparent organ of vision.

The aqueous from its origin in the ciliary epithelium passes through the pupil, fills the anterior chamber and drains through the trabecular meshwork in the angle of the anterior chamber. The flow is continuous although the quantity secreted fluctuates during the day.

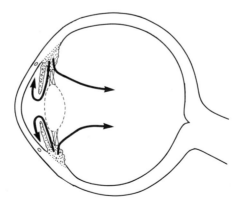

Fig. 12.1 When the aqueous fluid cannot leave the eye at the rate at which it enters, the eyeball becomes hard. When the pressure of the eyeball defeats the pressure of blood feeding the optic nerve head, the field of vision eventually succumbs and the patient does not realise what is happening because the central vision remains intact.

The circulation of aqueous may be blocked at:

1. the pupil – possibly by adhesions or a swollen lens
2. the trabecular meshwork in the angle of the anterior chamber, if the meshwork has been damaged.

   From the roll call of pathological causation – congenital, hereditary, traumatic, neoplastic, inflammatory and so on we can easily construct an unabridged catalogue of what might go wrong with the trabecular meshwork.

   In the absence of any demonstrable disease, we enter the territory of chronic simple glaucoma, where the trabecular meshwork malfunctions and as yet we really do not know why.

   'Simple' as part of a medical title is a code word meaning 'complex'. And no-one has yet explained why chronic glaucoma happens except that the disease would appear to be part of an ischaemic process affecting the whole eye.
3. the angle of the anterior chamber where the trabecular meshwork is normal but a pupil dilating in the presence of a shallow anterior chamber prevents the aqueous from getting there in the first place.

Glaucoma the process

Yet again we find the eye demonstrating a solitary response to a multiplicity of factors.

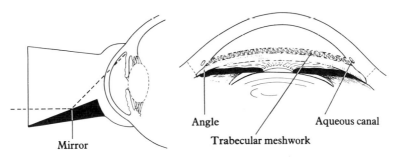

Fig. 12.2 An open angle seen through the gonioscope. Recession of the drainage angle through trauma or heavy deposition of pigment as in pigmentary glaucoma are examples of inflammation revealed by this technique.

In pathological terms, glaucoma the process can be regarded as a neuropathy of the optic nerve in which a raised intraocular pressure often plays a part.

In simplistic terms if the intraocular pressure is higher than the capillary pressure feeding the optic nerve then it effectively squeezes blood from the optic nerve head. This optic nerve head ischaemia has the following results:

1. A progressive defect in the visual field – the so-called arcuate scotoma which spreads from the normal blind spot. This blind spot is the non-seeing optic nerve head projected into the visual field. The arcuate loss curves nasally above and below fixation.
2. The cup in the optic nerve head increases in a vertical oval.
3. Because central vision remains unaffected, there is no subjective awareness of any danger.

Variations in the level of intraocular pressure

20 mmHg, as measured by the applanation tonometer, is taken as the upper limit of normal pressure. There are no sharp edges in nature and the range fluctuates from person to person and indeed in each person during the day, being highest in the morning. In some people the basal pressure is higher than 20 mmHg and may have to be accepted as being normal for them. We should avoid the temptation to call this raised pressure 'glaucoma'. It is much more reasonable to describe it as what it is – a raised intraocular pressure with no other recognizable features.

CHRONIC SIMPLE GLAUCOMA

Given our negligent acceptance of six different meanings, it can come as no surprise to learn that most patients actually use a seventh. They imagine 'glaucoma' as a composite condition combining the pain and haloes of angle closure with the visual loss of cataract and macular degeneration and the flashing lights of a retinal break. We would do everyone a service if we could define once and for all, not least to ourselves, what we mean when we talk of 'glaucoma'.

Chronic simple glaucoma is the name given to that neuropathy of the optic nerve which untreated leads on to 'glaucoma the process', the characteristics of which may safely tolerate repetition:

1.   arcuate scotomata
2.   extension of the round optic cup into a vertical oval
3.   (in most cases) an intraocular pressure that fluctuates throughout the day until it ends up permanently on the wrong side of normal.

Prevalence

One in 200 of the population over the age of 40 in the Western world have some evidence of chronic simple glaucoma.

Inheritance

Much needless anxiety is caused by the belief that the condition passes by dominant heredity. That someone's grandmother aged 85 is found to have chronic glaucoma does not mean that the entire family tree is suspect. Chronic glaucoma is a common condition and may well be passed through the recessive inheritance of a very common gene.

It has been stated that one in 10 of the close relatives of patients with chronic glaucoma will eventually go on to suffer the disorder themselves. Unfortunately this statement does not mention at what age. Clearly, chronic glaucoma established at 40 must raise a question mark over children once they reach the same age.

Chronic glaucoma starting for the first time at 80 does not call for regular testing of children, grandchildren or great grandchildren.

PATHOLOGY

The hard fact is that we do not know why chronic simple glaucoma happens. The exact cause, although thought to be somewhere in the trabecular meshwork, is not understood and it has, for that reason, been described by a wide range of synonyms. In practical terms we might reasonably imagine the trabecular meshwork to be like a garden sieve, clogging with debris as time passes.

There is more to it than that, because eyes with chronic glaucoma tend to succumb to the raised intraocular pressure, presumably because the optic nerve head is already trembling towards ischaemia and is vulnerable anyway.

When to refer

Until recently people with visual defects went to opticians who provided glasses. All visual loss was presumed to be due to refractive error and the notion that anything else might affect the eye never crossed anybody's mind.

Happily, after years of persuasion, all this has changed. People now go to optometrists who still provide glasses but who examine the eyes in great detail on the very wise principle that just because the eyes are seeing well does not mean that they are also healthy.

Unhappily, this very care, which is intended to save needless and futile work too late, is beginning to create a lot of work too early. Sophisticated field analysers are beginning to reveal areas of diminished sensitivity in the visual fields never dreamed of previously. The question is to know which are of consequence and which are not.

A similar question hangs over the significance of a raised intraocular pressure. Measured with the air puff tonometer it tends to read considerably higher than when measured by applanation. We must not assume that a raised pressure is a disease in itself. It is merely an observation. In the absence of:

1. field defects
2. cupping of the optic nerve head

a raised pressure has clearly not damaged the eye yet and may never do so.

Referral then, with a raised pressure alone, is not complete. The visual fields and optic nerve heads have to been considered also. Field defects in association with a fluctuating pressure are certainly the hallmark of chronic simple glaucoma. They do not, however, develop rapidly and in themselves they are not a justification for urgent referral.

The most sinister occult menace is possible occlusion of the central retinal vein. This common associate of chronic glaucoma is possibly more likely in the presence of other threats to the circulation from such as hypertension, diabetes or polycythaemia.

In the absence of any suggestion of circulatory incompetence, it would be reasonable to ask the optometrist to measure the limits of intraocular levels over a morning (phasing), because a wide swing between high in the morning and low by lunch time has been found to relate to the development of the other classic signs we associate with glaucoma. This also is an incidental reason why glaucoma clinics are not best conducted in the afternoon.

A pressure level, on the other hand, which starts with one level in the morning ending up with much the same at lunch time may very well be normal for that eye.

Eyes tend to behave in pairs. In the absence of any previous injury, pressures differing markedly between the eyes must be regarded with suspicion.

Not infrequently a second request for an ophthalmological opinion follows urgently on the heels of the first because the vision has appeared to decline further. The answer here is not an ophthalmologist's opinion but referral to the optometrist who suggested the opinion in the first place.

Unless the patient has suffered a central retinal vein occlusion, in which case the decline will be relatively sudden and severe, a slightly raised pressure can have no recognizable effect on the central vision – the only vision that patients know they have.

Raised pressure may certainly affect the field and the optic nerve head but it does not affect the macula and will not give rise to any new ophthalmic symptoms.

If the patient already has

1. field defects
2. cupping of the optic nerve head

then referral is obligatory. The degree of urgency depends on the severity of these findings.

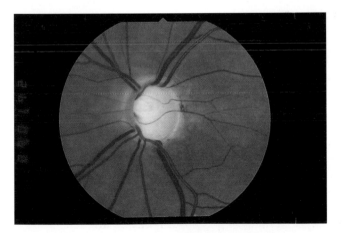

Fig. 12.3 Cupping of the optic nerve head – a classic sign of chronic simple glaucoma but the end result of any long period of raised intraocular pressure, whatever the cause.

In all other circumstances optometrists can continue the good work they have begun, examining patients in detail and continuing to examine them in detail until a suspicion of change necessitates referral to an eye surgeon.

Raised intraocular pressure

In most patients with chronic simple glaucoma, the first detectable sign would be an intraocular pressure that fluctuates throughout the day. This quiet fluctuation will not bring itself to our attention in any way and certainly not with pain.

The intraocular pressure, highest in the morning, will swing downwards over the day over a range of up to 5–6 mmHg. When this range swings beyond 5–6 mmHg then we should be suspicious.

Like all disease processes, chronic glaucoma has to begin sometime and what we find depends on when we start looking.

Visual field

The patches of reduced sensitivity progress to frank blind spots. These in turn enlarge and coalesce, quietly creeping towards fixation and outwards towards the edges of the visual field whilst the patient continues to read happily, unaware of impending doom.

In due course these so-called arcuate scotomata burst outwards and will involve the peripheral limits of the visual field.

Hand movement testing

Clearly in the early stages of the disease, testing the limits of vision with the hand will not pick up areas of reduced sensitivity within the margins of normal vision.

However, if the disease has gone unchecked, and unfortunately this happens all too frequently, defects when sufficiently advanced to be picked up by the hand will be noticed first of all on the nasal side.

The Damato test

This simple device allows us to search areas of the visual field where glaucoma defects are known to occur. It requires only a field testing chart and a pair of reading glasses (if worn) and good illumination (see Fig. 4.9, p.58).

Fundus

The optic nerve head betrays its submission to the disease by excavation of the normal round cup into a vertical oval.

LOW TENSION (NORMAL TENSION) GLAUCOMA

The two signs of 'glaucoma the process' –

1. classic field loss
2. classic disc cupping

develop with no intraocular pressure rise to explain them.

The given reason is that although the intraocular pressure is demonstrably low, the capillary blood pressure feeding the optic nerve head must be lower still. The diagnosis of low tension glaucoma can only be made when we have demonstrated that:

1. the intraocular pressure at all times over 24 hours is below the level accepted as normal (20 mmHg)
2. that no intracranial lesion, such as a pituitary adenoma or a parasellar meningioma, is simulating glaucoma field defects.

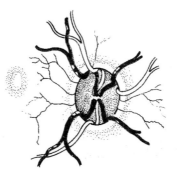

Fig. 12.4 Cupping of the optic nerve head. Once this degree of excavation is evident, field loss, particularly on the nasal side, can be picked up with the hands.

A lateral radiograph of the skull, although denounced now-adays as next to useless, can easily demonstrate the presence of an enlarged pituitary fossa.

Given its now reducing cost, a CT scan can certainly be taken as a more certain method of eliminating intracranial compressive disorders.

CENTRAL RETINAL VEIN OCCLUSION

This vascular catastrophe is one of the devastating associates of chronic glaucoma. Venous blood presumably flows with greater difficulty through a hard eye but the marvel is that it flows normally for so long in most circumstances.

Although any vascular episode must raise the possibility of

1. hypertension
2. diabetes
3. some blood dyscrasia

it also raises the likelihood of a raised intraocular pressure, which we should especially consider while going through the seven signs.

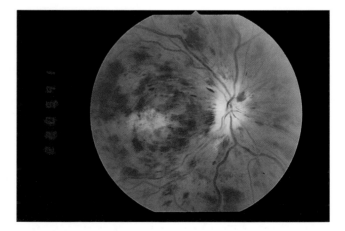

Fig. 12.5   Central retinal vein occlusion – the stormy sunset of central vision. Chronic simple glaucoma, hypertension, diabetes and hyperviscosity must be excluded as a matter of course.

MANAGEMENT

Treatment aims to bring down the intraocular pressure to a level where field defects become static. To eliminate the actual cause, which of course is the ideal of all medical treatment, is a despairing wish. A trabecular drain no longer drains properly and whatever is clogging it cannot be removed. However, the ill effects of blockage can be managed at least for a while with two guiding principles in mind:

1. to make the drain work more efficiently
2. to reduce aqueous production and thus reduce demands made on the drain.

The drugs in common use do not appear to follow any rational basis. Indeed it would appear that the success of each one raises more questions than it answers. The drugs in question seem to form a circle of autonomic contradiction:

1. inhibition of the
        sympathetic system
2. stimulation of the
        parasympathetic
        sympathetic

either singly or in combination, bring the pressure down by mechanisms that have not been explained yet.

Beta blockers

The beta-adrenergic receptor blocking agents also reduce intraocular pressure. Their action is primarily on inflow, but the outflow may be enhanced as well.

These drugs did not start off in happy association with the eye. Practolol was once a popular treatment for hypertension before its destructive effects on mucous membrane, including the conjunctiva, led to its withdrawal.

The first beta blocker used in ophthalmology was timolol but carteolol, betaxolol and levobunolol have now come on the scene and time will tell which is best. It may well be that none is best and that each will be favoured by different patients.

That they neither dilate nor constrict the pupil, nor drag on the peripheral retina, must recommend them. Unfortunately they have some less attractive features.

Reduction in the heart rate can be dangerous in patients with congestive cardiac failure and a tendency to bronchial spasm may be tipped into a frank attack of asthma. It is claimed that betaxolol as a selective beta blocker limits this latter risk.

Although patients may now see through a normal pupil, they may well not appreciate visual improvement if they cannot breathe whilst sliding further into congestive cardiac failure.

Despite all this talk of intraocular pressure control, at the end of the day, retention of the visual field depends on how much blood manages to squeeze into the optic nerve head against the pressure of the eye trying to squeeze it out. There is evidence to suggest a link with general vasospastic disease, which is marked by cold extremities that can sometimes become colder still when topical beta blockers find their way into the general circulation.

If the blood supply to the optic nerve head be similarly reduced, then the 'glaucoma the process' can continue to erode the visual field and cup the optic nerve head at pressure levels that might well seduce us all into believing that the drops are working successfully.

Different versions of these drugs come in different concentrations but all are used on a twice-daily basis except levobunolol which can be effective for 24 hours. There is probably no one drug that can be recommended over all the others, but when a beta blocker is to be used then one which causes asthma, bradycardia, cold feet and cold hands might reasonably be exchanged for one that does not – if it can be found.

Adrenaline

Adrenaline, stimulating both alpha and beta receptors, affects the inflow and the outflow. It is formulated as adrenaline proper or as dipivefrin – a so-called pro-drug which develops into adrenaline when instilled into the conjunctival sac.

Both dilate the pupil, weaken the reading focus and induce conjunctival injection. There is, however, a definite place for them in the management of glaucoma. In mild cases, they may well be strong enough to control the pressure on their own.

There are certain contraindications.

All adrenaline compounds have a harmful effect on the macula following cataract extraction and are thought to induce intraretinal macular oedema.

Because of their effects on the pupil they can clearly play no part in the management of acute angle closure where their administration could only augment the damage begun by the initial attack.

It is thought that, in combination with a beta blocker, although they certainly achieve the stated aim of reducing the intraocular pressure to a level that delights staff in the glaucoma clinic, they may also achieve the unstated aim of reducing the capillary blood flow through the optic nerve, thus allowing glaucoma the process to continue with beguiling malice.

Pilocarpine

Although this parasympathomimetic agent encourages the outflow of aqueous, a hundred years of research have told us no more than the fact that it happens. Various hypotheses have been offered. It has been suggested that the action is a mechanical one. The drug throws the muscle of accommodation into spasm and may pull open the meshwork to which it is attached. That is its only useful effect in chronic glaucoma. All the others are unwanted.

The same muscle of accommodation may pull off the retina to which it is attached. It throws the near focus into spasm; it reduces the size of the pupil and darkens the vision.

It also makes a patient who now cannot see properly wonder why everyone is so delighted with this management of a condition that had no symptoms before treatment was started.

However, the drug is, without question, effective and can be given up to four times a day. A 1% solution probably does as much good as a stronger solution, and probably considerably less harm.

Acetazolamide

This drug, now discarded as a diuretic, has regained a place in medicine by the very significant effect it has on aqueous production.

Although suspect from time to time because of potassium loss or metabolic acidosis, it may have a place in the treatment of those whose fingers are still too stiff to manipulate bottles, or whose memories are too wayward to remember.

Nausea, finger tingling, renal calculi and frank psychosis may force us to abandon acetazolamide, and it should not be forgotten that it was not used as the original diuretic for nothing.

A maximum dosage of 1 g daily may be tolerated for a short while. Half that dosage, or less, may be tolerated for longer, and indeed may have to be.

Intolerance of acetazolamide sometimes leads to the prescription of dichlorphenamide in the usually mistaken hope that it will cause fewer ill effects.

Surgery

If, by all these measures, progression of chronic field loss is halted then regular examination (eventually every 6 months) is required to ensure that the arrest is maintained. Should field loss continue despite maximum medical therapy, then the decision edges towards surgery.

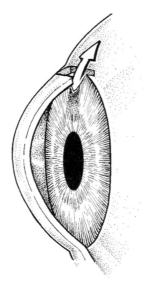

Fig. 12.6   The principles of glaucoma surgery. A hole is cut from the anterior chamber into the subconjunctival space, allowing aqueous to bypass the damaged trabecular meshwork. The peripheral iridectomy nullifies the effects of blockage at the pupil.

Nowadays this reluctance to operate is giving way to a reluctance not to. Once it is evident that medical control is losing the battle, then there is nothing to be gained by continuing the same battle. Indeed there is much to be lost – by the patient (not by the doctor), for it has been shown that the drugs given to reduce the pressure actually induce fibrosis in the very areas where it is not wanted. Surgery aims to drain off aqueous through a permanent fistula into the sub-conjunctival space. Such a channel is unnatural and the fibrotic response by young eyes and by African eyes may close off the neatest surgical drain.

It has been shown recently that a cytotoxic agent like mitomycin C, if applied over the surgical field deep to the conjunctiva, can prevent this natural response from bringing about yet another surgical failure just when success is particularly desired.

Fortunately, older eyes where the healing response is more feeble and where these operations are most often required do not close off the drain site completely. But even if successful, surgery can upset the aqueous balance which in turn upsets the lens which in turn does the only thing it can by becoming opaque.

As with all surgical manoeuvres the possible complications of operating have to be balanced against the greater complications of not operating. Glaucoma is one of these impossible conditions were doctor and patient are frequently at loggerheads. To start with, people go along to their opticians in search of new lenses for their old frames and end up (even today) with pilocarpine. We tell them that they are doing well, that they will continue to see well in the future and they retort that they cannot see now.

For that reason there is much to be said for keeping pilocarpine up the sleeve – possibly for ever. We must find a regime that pleases the patient and pleases us. It is pointless to turn someone's life into a series of brief intervals between drops which darken the vision just as it was beginning to recover from the effects of the last treatment.

Molteno valve

When fibrosis neutralizes the effect of surgery or is expected to do so in particular patients, solid silicone rubber can be implanted into the subconjunctival space and the anterior chamber to maintain the surgical fistula.

Further fibrosis has to be suppressed with systemic corticosteroids and occasionally cytotoxic drugs. Once the patient has navigated these rapids there is still the darkening cataract, the effects of which have to be distinguished from the darkening effects of the glaucoma process itself.

WHEN TO TREAT

When does a raised pressure become 'glaucoma'? This is one of the hardest questions to answer. Authorities differ, some treating it as 'glaucoma' whilst others, in the absence of cupping and field defects, call it 'ocular hypertension'.

A long-established tradition has certainly been to await the development of unequivocal glaucoma signs. This is all very well, provided the signs are cupping and field defects, but not very well if the first sign is a central retinal vein occlusion.

It is conceivable that this waiting approach is a relic of the days when pilocarpine was the first line of treatment. It is quite understandable that patients perhaps preferred the risk of possible visual loss from glaucoma to definite visual loss from pilocarpine.

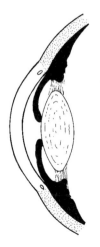

Fig. 12.7   The tendency to angle closure is a shape until something happens. The sympathetic pulls the pupil open and backwards against the lens. Pupil block builds up aqueous behind the iris, which bulges forwards and blocks the drainage meshwork.

ACUTE ANGLE CLOSURE

That acute angle closure, by tradition, is also given the title primary glaucoma might at first suggest yet another inexplicable disaster couched in words without meaning. Happily this is not so. The cause lies in the shape of the eye:

1. a shallow anterior chamber
2. a narrow angle.

The precipitating factor is a pupil dilating under the influence of:

1. reduced illumination
2. sympathetic stimulation
3. some factors as yet unidentified.

Until this happens, we are facing not a disease but a shape. The acute attack is quite clearly secondary to a collection of circumstances made significant by that shape and is best described as acute angle closure rather than acute glaucoma.

It is commonly believed that acute angle closure is but chronic simple glaucoma with pain and haloes. This is manifest nonsense. There is no connection between the two unless someone is unfortunate to have both.

The eye with the dangerous shape is long-sighted, with an anterior chamber too shallow for safe dilatation of the pupil. The advance of middle-age exaggerates this shallowness by a forward movement of the iris–lens diaphragm.

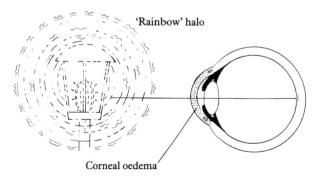

'Rainbow' halo

Corneal oedema

Fig. 12.8   The sodden cornea, like the sky after rain, breaks light into a ring of spectral colours. Any halo without these colours is not caused by angle closure.

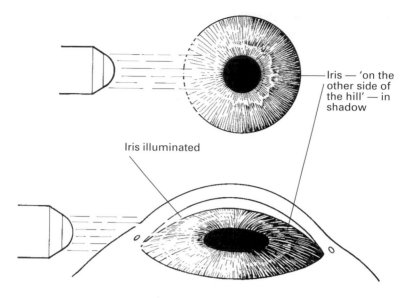

Iris — 'on the other side of the hill' — in shadow

Iris illuminated

Fig. 12.9   The eclipse test is one of the essential signs. An eye with so shallow an anterior chamber may not have its pupil dilated. All others may.

Extreme long sight has two further associates – thick glasses that obscure distant objects to all but those for whom they were prescribed, and not infrequently a convergent squint dating from childhood.

However, simple dilatation of the pupil is not the whole story. Activation of the dilator fibres – innervated by the sympathetic – drags the iris back against the lens. Aqueous, failing to pass the pupil, pushes the peripheral iris forwards, where in a small eye it will suddenly occlude the trabecular meshwork. It is not that the pupil dilates, but how it dilates.

Like a character in a Greek tragedy, the eye appears to be at peace with its fatal flaw. Then the harbingers of doom issue their brief warnings. There are fleeting elevations of pressure. A sodden corneal stroma breaks light up into rainbow haloes and blurs the vision. Pain in the forehead can be mistaken for 'evening migraine' Unlike a Greek tragedy , the final disaster need not be inevitable.

It is passed from text to text that likely victims are edgy, middle-aged women, whose anterior chambers have shallowed sufficiently to allow their draining mechanism to succumb to their purposeless fretting. Perhaps the time has come to abandon this stereotype. There are just as many edgy, middle-aged men.

The acute attack

This is one of the three major red eyes. Inflammation dominates around the corneo-scleral limbus, and which of the three serious red eyes it is will be revealed by the seven signs.

1. *Central vision – distance*: blurred.
2. *Central vision –* near: blurred.
3. *Field vision*: a very steamy cornea might blur this as well.
4. *Cornea*: oedematous, with an appearance reminiscent of water hosing down a fishmonger's window.
5. *Pupil* (if visible): fixed and half dilated.
6. *Anterior chamber* (if visible): shallow; that of fellow eye also shallow.
7. *Intraocular pressure*: eye rock-hard.

MANAGEMENT

Problems

1. The high pressure will blind the eye unless something is done rapidly.
2. The longer the attack, the more likely the trabecular damage.
3. Aqueous continually secreted – cannot get out.

Action

1. Aqueous production must be reduced immediately. Acetazolamide (500 mg) has to be given, if necessary by intravenous injection. It acts quicker this way (it is also much more expensive) and in a nauseated patient may be obligatory.
2. Because the pupil is dilated it must be constricted – intensive topical pilocarpine.
3. If pilocarpine fails to reduce the pupil, then the next step must be to reduce the extracellular fluid with an intravenous infusion of mannitol: 250–500 ml of a 20% solution; administration of any concentration should not be considered

in patients with congestive cardiac failure or pulmonary oedema.

As the drug appears to drain the body into the bladder, acute retention of urine may take the place of acute retention of aqueous. As long as these possible side effects are anticipated, it is sometimes the only effective medical way of bringing a recalcitrant attack of acute angle closure to heel.

The tendency is bilateral, and the pupil-reducing qualities of pilocarpine, perhaps twice daily, can protect the fellow eye in the short term. In the long term, however, pilocarpine will not do. It can block aqueous flow at the pupil and actually increase the danger of acute angle closure.

Surgery

Once the pressure is reduced, surgery should prevent subsequent elevation.

A peripheral iridectomy – a hole cut in the iris near its root – allows aqueous to bypass the pupil between its source in the ciliary body and its outflow at the drainage angle.

A peripheral iridectomy is certainly the operation of choice for the fellow eye. If the attack has been prolonged, simply allowing the aqueous to reach the drainage angle will be useless because the drain, damaged eventually by the raised pressure, will no longer be draining.

A peripheral iridectomy will certainly allow the aqueous to make it to the angle; an external fistula, as for chronic glaucoma, will then let it out of the eye.

THE ASYMPTOMATIC SHALLOW ANTERIOR CHAMBER

A shallow anterior chamber alone is not enough to justify interference, because the treatment is surgical, and surgery must be justified.

Not all anterior chambers with positive eclipse tests are dangerous. But all that are dangerous have a positive eclipse. The riddle is to know which are dangerous.

First of all we can look at the gap between the iris and the trabecular meshwork through an angled mirror and a contact lens. This technique is known as gonioscopy. This will tell us the gap is narrow, which we suspected anyway. Sometimes it is not as narrow as we imagined.

It is at this point that theory breaks down in the face of reality and tests to 'prove' that an angle can close never mimic nature. The best they can do is dilate the pupil one way or another whilst we look for a rising pressure.

The so-called provocative tests

Dark room test

The patient, well furnished with explanations, is left in a darkened room for about an hour, after which any rise in intraocular pressure is noted.

Physiology is well harnessed here because we are testing the two elements thought to be directly related to angle closure – relaxation of the sphincter plus active stimulation of the sympathetic dilator. The first comes from absent light, the second from sheer terror at what might be happening. A negative response leaves us in the dark also.

Drug-induced attack

A dangerous anterior chamber may continue to appear innocent when simple mydriasis fails to block the flow of aqueous in a vain attempt to ape the genuine catastrophe. If the pressure does go up with dilatation of the pupil then the answer is a bilateral peripheral iridectomy. If the pressure does not go up the answer may still be a bilateral peripheral iridectomy but not necessarily immediately. Research is going on at the moment to determine the value of iridotomy with the YAG laser – a cold beam which explodes a hole in the iris at the point of impact. As we might guess, such an explosion is not without its dangers. Pigment dispersal can block the trabecular sieve even more effectively than the postulated debris of chronic simple glaucoma.

Before we congratulate ourselves, we have to recognize that a positive 'test' may have brought about an acute closure of the angle that might otherwise never have happened.

It is possible that the wisest recourse is to explain about haloes and blurring of vision at dusk and leave nature to do what she will.

INFANTILE GLAUCOMA (BUPHTHALMOS)

Developmental remnants lingering in the angle have the usual
solitary effect in raising intraocular pressure. The growing eye
adds another feature of its own and grows more than it ought to
because the inner pressure makes it stretch.

SECONDARY RISE OF PRESSURE

When an eye hardens in response to any other recognizable
agency, we use the term secondary glaucoma. It would be pleasing to exchange the word here for secondary pressure rise or some
such synonym. The causes lie anywhere along the pathway of
aqueous from the pupil to the drainage meshwork in the anterior
chamber angle. The list of common pathology can provide the
causes which will include:

1. congenital malfunction of the angle
2. traumatic scarring of the meshwork
3. iritic debris in the meshwork
4. diabetic new vessel formation at the iris root
5. iritic debris anywhere
6. iritic adhesions at the pupil.

When the drama of the primary condition has settled any secondary rise of pressure, if unsuspected, may set in motion glau-

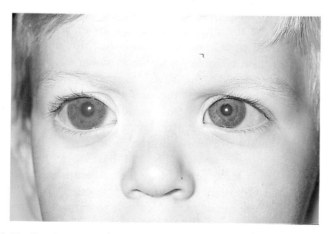

Fig. 12.10 Buphthalmos – infantile glaucoma. The raised intraocular pressure
stretches the sclera, producing a large, watering, photophobic eye.

coma the process' and destroy the visual field as silently and effectively as happens in chronic simple glaucoma.

To foresee and forestall this wanton destruction, we must always think aqueous and ask ourselves – has something happened to obstruct the aqueous flow?

MANAGEMENT

Acute conditions like iritis produce an acute pressure rise. The scars of trauma could affect the eye long after the original injury has settled, and indeed be forgotten.

Management is just a variation on the old theme. It splits up into medical, surgical, short term or long term.

If the pressure is high the problem is urgent. If the pressure is only moderate, then we can take our time.

Sometimes the primary condition takes precedence, sometimes it does not. However, as with chronic simple glaucoma, the first step in treating a raised pressure is to think of it.

SUMMARY

The word glaucoma is used in six different ways:

1. a pathological process resulting in field loss and disc cupping
2. any rise of intraocular pressure
3. pressure rising as a sequel to some recognized condition
4. the named disease chronic simple glaucoma
5. the named disease acute angle closure
6. the named disease infantile glaucoma.

'Glaucoma the process' is the only correct use but the named condition of chronic simple glaucoma is too well established to be readily abandoned.

All pressure rises are secondary to something. In chronic simple glaucoma, the pressure rises secondary to nothing obvious. The eye is ischaemic and some malfunction of the trabecular sieve and possibly of the blood supply to the optic nerve head contribute to the development of glaucoma the process.

Low or normal tension glaucoma is chronic simple glaucoma with no high pressure to account for it.

Intracranial space occupying lesions such as a pituitary adenoma or a paracellular meningioma can compress the visual pathways into a simulation of classic field defects. It is not unknown for patients to be treated for chronic low tension glaucoma when the real cause could have been revealed by a lateral radiograph of the skull or in greater detail by a CT scan.

It must be remembered that a quiet rise of intraocular pressure can destroy the visual fields in the absence of any symptoms, because central vision is unaffected.

Acute angle closure is secondary to a shallow anterior chamber. Until it happens, this tendency is not a disease; it is a shape.

MANAGEMENT

If the intraocular pressure is shown to be damaging the visual field, then it has to be reduced by:

1. topical medications
2. oral medications
3. filtration surgery
4. all three.

In acute angle closure, the pressure must be reduced urgently. Surgery is always required to bypass the obstruction to the aqueous flow within the small eye and possibly outside if the drainage meshwork has been damaged by the raised pressure.

Secondary rise in intraocular pressure – the cause or the pressure itself, whichever is more urgent, should be dealt with first. A high pressure usually takes precedence. What the rise was secondary to, may be forgotten in the mists of youth when the reserves of drainage concealed a silent menace for the future.

13. Diabetes and the eye

Diabetic complications within the eye must rank in the Western World as one of the most common causes of irreversible blindness today. They are possibly less momentous in the Third World where even more serious causes of blindness remain to be dealt with. Complications are more likely to develop in patients who have had diabetes for some time. Insulin-dependent diabetics generally have 5 years grace, but after 15 years of diabetic life, some 90% of them will be carrying some evidence of diabetic eye disease.

Non-insulin-dependent diabetics, on the other hand, may not even know when their disease started. They may, in fact, not know they have diabetes at all, until visual decline sparks off a series of medical investigations that seem curiously unconnected with the eye.

Although ocular complications become more common the longer the disease goes on, other factors influence their development.

Control

It has been suspected for a long time, but is now increasingly proven, that a reduction in the incidence and severity of ocular dysfunction is almost directly related to tight control. This involves regular urine testing by the patient, the efficacy of which can be monitored by regular estimates of blood sugar.

A certain amount of glucose is bound to haemoglobin. In the non-diabetic population, this glycosylated haemoglobin (haemoglobin A_1) should account for some 5.5–8.0% of the total. The exact level varies from laboratory to laboratory.

In poorly controlled diabetics, on the other hand, the figure can rise above 20%. Proper attention to diet and to the urine sugar is parallelled by a decline in the levels of this glycosylated haemoglobin.

Hypertension

It is one of the ironies of life that a blood pressure higher than it ought to be actually reduces the general flow of blood throughout the body. Since the essential damage of diabetes is to the small blood vessels, the two conditions combine to accelerate the ill effects of each other.

Alcohol

Abuse of alcohol – a fashionable phrase – is also considered to have a malign influence. What is abuse and what is being good company will be interpreted against the intake of the medical observer. The young everywhere are capable of consuming vast quantities of alcohol as a matter of course and 1 in every 100 will be diabetic.

Tobacco

This human solace brought from the New World by Walter Ralegh, denounced by James VI and I in his *Counterblaste to Tobacco* must now sadly be withdrawn from the list of (socially) acceptable poisons. The quick drag to 'calm the nerves' has probably resulted in even more things to worry about. Quite apart from what it does to the lungs, its restriction of blood flow everywhere can be of no added benefit, particularly to a diabetic.

Although it is generally accepted that attention to:

— control
— hypertension
— reduction of alcohol intake
— abandonment of tobacco

clearly reduces the complications of diabetes, recent work would suggest that in time all diabetics will display some evidence of eye disease if their diabetes goes on for long enough.

EFFECTS OF DIABETES ON THE EYE

The essential lesion in diabetes is in the wall of the small blood vessels – all over the body but only in the eye is its evil so instantly apparent.

Microaneurysm

The weakened walls of the small vessels bulge in places and round red blobs scattered throughout the fundus are the first sign that diabetes is affecting the eye.

Haemorrhage

The weakened vessels have a tendency to leak blood into the retina. Blood appears red, but its shape will be dictated by its position:

1. deep haemorrhages are round – because the deep layers are tightly packed
2. surface haemorrhages are flame-shaped – following the nerve-fibre pattern
3. preretinal haemorrhages form a fluid level between the retina and the vitreous
4. vitreal haemorrhages are restrained only by the limits of the vitreal cavity.

Exudates

Given such vascular incompetence, it is not surprising to find oedema collecting within the retina itself. The ensuing damage to retinal tissue releases lipids, which are picked up by macrophages. These cells, gorged with cholesterol, become visible as yellow-white, hard exudates.

Ischaemia

Venous changes

Distortion and dilatation of the retinal veins, which might not attract much attention, are the first clear sign that the retinal blood supply is not coping with the demands.

Cotton-wool spots

Once known as soft exudates, cotton-wool spots are another unequivocal sign of even more severe retinal ischaemia. It is simplistic to regard them as retinal infarcts. Present thinking ascribes them to axonal transport material accumulating because axonal flow has come to a halt.

It was not uncommon in the past to see on case records a description of 'soft exudates hardening'. This of course is nonsense. Soft exudates which, of course, are not exudates at all, but better known as cotton-wool spots, do not harden; they disappear. By dropping the term soft exudate permanently, we can eliminate at least one misconception.

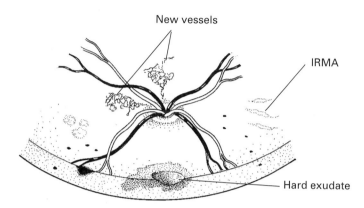

Fig. 13.1 Diabetic retinopathy on the high road to disaster. Tight control might well have delayed this picture. The severity of the diabetes is not relevant.

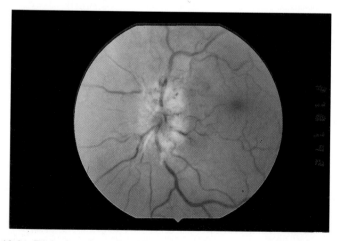

Fig. 13.2 Diabetic retinopathy. The more moderate changes are marked by variation in venous calibre, higher exudates and round, red eye areas which may be either blot haemorrhages or microaneurysms.

Intraretinal microvascular abnormalities (IRMA)

Intraretinal dilated capillaries can be picked up with the ophthalmoscope. A green filter, which eliminates the red of the choroid, makes it possible to outline these elongated dilatations as black against a pale-green background. Together with venous changes, extensive intraretinal haemorrhages and cotton-wool spots, they combine to indicate that the retina has now entered the preproliferative phase – they are a sort of prologue setting the scene for the tragedy about to unfold.

Proliferation

Severe hypoxia stimulates the retina to seek other sources of oxygen. New blood vessels now enter to remedy this want. However, instead of oxygen to the retina, they raise the great danger of blood in the vitreous, to which they are adherent.

It is not unusual for the diabetic vitreal gel to collapse and shrink, tearing the new vessels in the process. Blood is released into the space vacated by the collapsing gel, or actually into the gel itself.

The haemorrhage appears to stimulate fibrosis which, although possibly a misguided attempt at healing, can in its own right be as ruinous as the haemorrhage. A fine membrane adherent to the

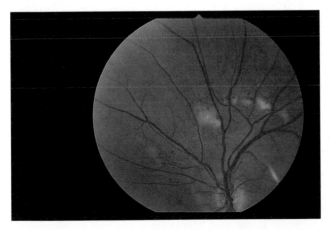

Fig. 13.3   Diabetic retinopathy. The advance into severe ischaemia continues with cotton wool spots, obvious as fluffy smudges, and new blood vessels sprouting from the optic nerve head.

retinal surface may wrinkle and pucker like kitchen 'clingfilm', pulling the retina into all manner of patterns and indeed often pulling it off altogether.

Although people still talk of background and proliferative retinopathy, the distinction is meaningless, as are attempts to grade the process with numbers. Any diabetic retinal change, no matter how bland it looks at one visit, is capable of threatening sight before the next.

Intravenous fluorescein angiography

Sodium fluorescein – the same dye used to pick up deficiencies in the corneal epithelium – can be equally informative about retinal function.

Injected into an arm vein, it passes throughout the body and can be photographed as it passes through the eye.

Irradiation with blue light induces fluorescence of the dye as it passes through the choroidal and retinal circulations.

The dye, collecting where it should not and lingering when it ought not, can reveal gaps and cracks in the ocular layers, together with leaks, stasis and closure in the fundal circulation.

Macula

Central visual loss is most commonly brought about by macular oedema. This results from capillary incompetence, both leakage and transport of the blood that remains intravascular. In addition the pigment epithelium upon which the neuro-retina depends for continued health becomes defective in some as yet unexplained way.

Loss of macular function therefore may be related to:

1. focal patches of oedema
2. diffusely disseminated oedema
3. ischaemia.

Pregnancy

As might be expected, the fluctuating volume of body fluid with its effect on blood sugar and blood pressure can accelerate the progression of serious retinopathy.

MANAGEMENT

Affection of macula

At present laser photocoagulation is the only treatment that has proved to be beneficial for macular oedema – and that not always.

The therapeutic aim is to bring about a resolution of the intraretinal oedema and absorption of hard exudates. However, once hard exudates have damaged the macular receptors eliminating them does not restore function.

Successful treatment depends on early recognition and prompt intervention with the laser. This of course raises a diagnostic dilemma because laser photocoagulation is potentially destructive in its own right. Early recognition implies that the central vision is still functioning at a reasonable level. The dilemma is to decide which is more dangerous, to leave the central vision possibly to decline or possibly not to decline or to interfere with the laser possibly to preserve central vision only to hasten its ultimate dissolution.

Proliferation

Something more radical with the laser is necessary here. It was observed that diabetics with spontaneous widespread chorioretinal scarring, from whatever cause, tended not to develop proliferative eye disease.

It was further observed that inducing such scars with some form of coagulation had the same effect.

The present fashion is to induce these scars with the argon laser. Theory presumes that such widespread scarring balances the oxygen consumed by the retina with the oxygen available to the retina, thus reducing the stimulus to the formation of new blood vessels.

The argon laser produces burns in the pigment retina, which engulf the adjacent cells of the neuro-retina – the part supplied by the choroid. It is thought that the oxygen from the choroid can then diffuse more easily and in quantities that are now adequate for the pigment epithelium and the outer retinal layers.

It should be remembered that the laser is light and has to travel through clear ocular structures. If the structures are not clear, because of either cataract or vitreal haemorrhage, then photocoagulation is impossible.

fibre layer of the retina because of partial absorption at that level. Such damage can be reduced by using argon green, with the blue wave-lengths illuminated.

Lasers, particularly those produced from argon gas, are not machines that can be turned on and off, day in day out without showing some degree of temperament. They require a special light source, plumbed-in water cooling or noisy air cooling and the regular services of a skilled engineer to keep them in active service. For those reasons all over the world we find units provided with argon lasers to keep them up to date with the latest technology but sadly not all of them are working.

The next few years will bring a new generation of solid-state lasers to produce whatever wave-length we consider effective and more likely to flourish in the absence of regular maintenance. With such qualities it can only be a matter of time before the argon laser is superseded completely.

Vitrectomy

Many eyes that in the past used to end up blind and painful can now be salvaged. It has become possible in recent years to do the unthinkable and enter the posterior cavity of the eye. A probe

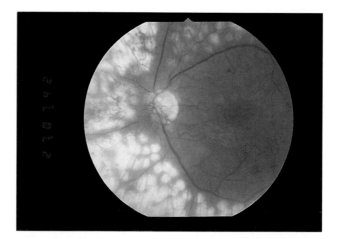

Fig. 13.4   Treated diabetic retinopathy – widespread chorioretinal scars brought about by argon laser photocoagulation. The characteristic feature is their distribution. Each one on its own has all the other features that make all chorioretinal scars look the same.

slipped into the vitreous, between the rectus muscle insertion and the lens, can cut and aspirate actual vitreal strands, or vitreal blood that refuses to clear away.

The guillotined fragments are sucked up the probe in a solution of balanced salt, which enters the eye as quickly as the cutter removes it.

The same entry point now allows the direct obliteration of bleeding vessels with underwater diathermy. Intravitreal traction bands can be cut with microscissors. The pre-retinal 'clingfilm' can be peeled away. Retinae detached by traction can be re-attached. And if opacities prevent the passage of the laser through the clear media, it can be delivered from within the eye through a microprobe.

Such intervention becoming with increasing usage standard rather than heroic, has brought hope to diabetics and their medical attendants.

Doubtless in time further biochemical advance will make vitrectomy as dated as pituitary ablation.

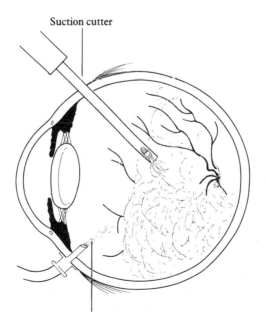

Suction cutter

Balanced salt inflow to maintain ocular volume

Fig. 13.5   Following vitrectomy, the eye can survive with balanced salt solution in place of vitreous, which can be removed on account of persistent haemorrhage or fibrosis.

OTHER PROBLEMS

Although such dramatic obliteration of vision can dominate the clinical picture, there are other ocular calamities.

Diabetics, more prone to vascular accidents anywhere in the body, have a higher incidence of occlusion of the central retinal vein and the central retinal artery than do comparable age groups in the non-diabetic population.

Diabetic eyes bleed during surgery when other eyes would not, and they tend to respond with much greater postoperative inflammation than other eyes might.

New vessel formation is not confined to the retina. It can insinuate itself into the drainage angle, creeping over the root of the iris and the trabecular meshwork with a catastrophic and usually irreversible effect on the intraocular pressure.

Cataract at an earlier age than usual concludes this catalogue of misfortune.

Until we discover the metabolic magic bullet, the first course of action for a diabetic is to accept the limitations on self-indulgence imposed by the need for rigid control. The second is to find a physician who is prepared to scrutinize the fundi through the dilated pupils at least once a year and sometimes more often. The third is to find an eye surgeon to liaise with the physician to form a team upon which effective total management depends.

SUMMARY

After 15 years of diabetic life, 90% of insulin-dependent patients have some evidence of diabetic eye disease.

Non-insulin-dependent patients may present with severe ocular and cardiovascular problems, because their diabetes appears mild enough to be ignored.

In time all diabetics appear to be affected.

Damage to the small blood vessels produces the ophthalmic appearances:

1. microaneurysms
2. round haemorrhages
3. hard exudates
4. venous abnormalities
5. cotton-wool spots
6. IRMA
7. new vessel formation.

Prognostic indicators

— duration of diabetes
— hypertension
— alcohol abuse
— smoking
— proteinuria
— glycosylated haemoglobins
— pregnancy.

Laser photocoagulation may:

1. clear intraretinal oedema before it leads on to permanent macular dysfunction
2. prevent the progression of proliferative retinopathy by the induction of widespread chorioretinal scars (panretinal photocoagulation).

Vitrectomy increases the surgical repertoire where proliferation has involved the vitreal cavity.

14. Hypertension and the eye

The response of the eye to hypertension, like so much else, can be made incomprehensible over several chapters. Yet, as might be predicted, the retina and its vessels reply in a very uncomplicated way, influenced only by three elements:

1. the state of the blood vessels before hypertension
2. the rate of development of hypertension
3. the ultimate level of the hypertension.

STATE OF THE BLOOD VESSELS

In childhood, the retinal venules and arterioles are of equal width. Both are well-endowed with elastic tissue and the arterioles also with muscle. They glisten regularly in the light of an ophthalmoscope.

As the blood pulses normally through these retinal vessels over the years, both the elastic and the muscles are in due course

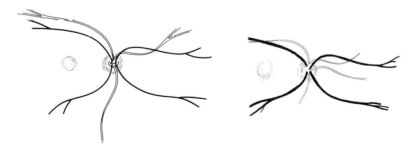

Fig. 14.1   (**a**) In a child, the arterioles and venules are of equal width and the general background of the retina glistens. (**b**) In an adult, the arterioles are narrower than the venules. The background loses the sparkle of youth.

replaced by fibrous material which dulls the glistening arteriolar reflexes.

In addition the calibre of the arterioles becomes slightly reduced and the shifting highlights of the young retina give way to a dry, coarse mottling. When the age of decline arrives, these fibrotic changes may, without offence, be given the name involutionary sclerosis. The fundamental point is that the vessels of the young eye, full of elastic tissue and muscle, will behave very differently from the rigid fibrotic vessels of an older eye when threatened with hypertension.

RATE OF DEVELOPMENT OF HYPERTENSION

When blood pressure moves into the pathological range it may:

1. rise slowly and moderately
2. rise swiftly to unrecordable levels.

The response of the eye is not the same in each case.

Gradual moderate rise (less than 200/120 mmHg)

The ageing eye

Involutionary changes are exaggerated. Any muscle remaining in the arterioles goes into spasm. The fibrotic stems remain very much as they were or even dilate somewhat. There is no need to complicate further this origin of arteriolar calibre variation.

These irregularities can be seen with the ophthalmoscope. Should the ophthalmoscopic light begin to fail, artefacts which masquerade as significant features can be picked up also. The often described shift in the arteriolar reflex from silver to copper is not a sign of ophthalmic disease but one of battery failure. None the less, it keeps turning up in textbook after textbook like a rich aunt that no one dare exclude from the wedding list.

Differences can now be seen developing at the arteriovenous (A/V) crossings. Thickening of the arteriolar wall is obvious only where it passes over or under a venule and gives the illusion of actual compression.

These A/V changes can be taken as the point where pathological evidence of hypertension is taking over from physiological evidence of passing time.

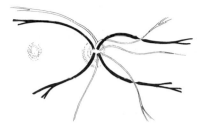

Fig. 14.2   Nipping at the arteriovenous crossing is the first evidence on the eye of a raised blood pressure. The first evidence of hypertension must surely be picked up with the sphygmomanometer.

The youthful eye

Exposed to a languid and moderate rise of blood pressure, young vessels protect themselves with involutionary patterns which, although acceptable at 60, must be regarded as pathological at 20. We should then not be surprised to see A/V nipping.

Both the old eye and the young eye now go on to the next stage in the process with haemorrhages, flamed over the surface of the retina in the pattern of the superficial layers. Lipids from disintegrating nerve tissue settles usually in the macula following the pattern of retinal fibres in a star shape around the macular hollow.

Rapid rise in blood pressure (greater than 200/120 mmHg)

The ageing eye

All the changes described above will develop but with greater speed and indeed occasionally with quite savage rapidity. Age brings its consolations and the presence of involutionary change actually protects the retinal vessels against severe elevations of pressure.

The youthful eye

Vessels without the protection of involution suffer grievously. Severe and uniform spasm of the arteriole is a prelude to actual blockage and retinal necrosis. The ischaemic retina becomes swollen and functionless.

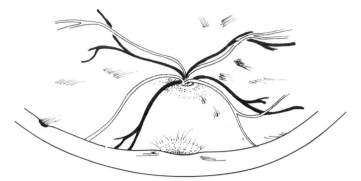

Fig. 14.3   Arteriovenous crossing changes, scattered flame-shaped haemorrhages and a macular star are findings classically associated with hypertension, though hopefully prevented by adequate systemic treatment.

Cotton-wool spots indicating acute retinal ischaemia then appear in both age groups. Haemorrhages present in simple hypertension will, of course, become more florid and indeed may burst into the vitreous.

Finally the optic nerve head takes part and swells into a state of papilloedema (malignant hypertension).

GRADING

There have been several attempts to produce a numerical shorthand for these developments and that most commonly used was described by Keith & Wagener:

Stage 1:   slight narrowing or sclerosis of arterioles

Stage 2:   more pronounced arteriole or calibre variations
A/V nipping
scattered flame shaped haemorrhages
the occasional hard exudate

Stage 3:   we are now into the range of severe hypertensive change, including all the above together with
1. pronounced haemorrhages
2. scattered exudates
3. cotton wool patches
4. marked retinal oedema

Stage 4:   all the above, together with papilloedema (choked disc).

Although this grading has its uses, dangers lurk in the shadows when we talk of one grade to someone who imagines we are talking about a completely different grade. Although it might take a little longer there is a lot to be said for describing what we see.

COMPLICATIONS

Occlusion of the central retinal artery

Interruption in the arterial flow leads rapidly to total retinal infarction. The retina, normally transparent, clouds into opacity, except at the macula where the cherry-red choroid can be seen through the macular hollow.

In time the retina becomes transparent again. The red reflex returns but alas the vision does not. The optic nerve head does not regain its glow but rather whitens into ischaemic optic atrophy.

Occlusion of the central retinal vein

The disc is swollen and haemorrhages dominate the appearance of an equally swollen retina. Should the oxygen supply be compromised, and it is not always, the eye may respond as it does in diabetes, with new blood vessels sprouting out over the retina and creeping over the iris root into the drainage angle where it may bring aqueous outflow to a merest trickle, turning the eye into a visually useless ball of pain and redness.

Action

The essential question is: how do we identify those eyes that will go on to develop this neovascular rise in pressure (rubeotic glaucoma) from those that will not?

Certain features indicate ischaemia:

1. severely diminished central vision
2. languid or absent constriction of the pupil in response to light
3. retinal capillary closure demonstrated by fluorescein
    angiography if wide scatter of retinal haemorrhages allow this.

The trouble is, that although many eyes with positive signs of ischaemia go on to develop a neovascular pressure rise, not all of them do and it would appear to be brutal to subject them all to widespread laser photocoagulation for two simple reasons:

1. laser coagulation is not bland and can severely restrict the peripheral vision
2. there are quite enough diabetics to occupy our lasers full time.

We then are faced with the philosophical question – is laser damage to the visual field when it was not necessary less acceptable than an intractable neovascular pressure rise when it might have been avoided! This question is being debated earnestly at the moment and a wide multicentre trial under way in the United States may well provide an answer in the not very distant future.

In the past it was customary to do nothing, whether necessary or not, because there was nothing that could be done. Patients were instructed to return to hospital in 3 months. If they returned in pain they would be told they had the '100-day glaucoma' (yet another meaning for that word). That everyone seemed to know what would happen and when it would happen somehow gave an air of wisdom to their total inability to do anything about it.

As for the time-scale, stained with blood, 100 days passed between Napoleon's escape from Elba and the final eclipse of the empire at Waterloo. As for the swollen veins, we need look no further than the Congress of Vienna, where droves of elderly statesmen, fully occupied in doing not very much, choked in horror at the news that the Emperor of the French was once more in Paris.

Hypertension is not the only cause of central retinal vein occlusion. It is an equally frequent associate of chronic simple glaucoma, of which it may be a presenting sign, and of diabetes.

Vitreal haemorrhage

Fragile capillaries rupturing into the vitreal cavity sometimes clear briefly to reveal no actual source of bleeding before a fresh flood of haemorrhage obscures the fundus once again.

We must remember that there are other causes of bleeding into the vitreous, not least diabetes, to which we may add a retinal break or a retinal break complicated by retinal detachment.

MANAGEMENT

Hypertension in the young is not usually 'essential', which means that a cause can usually be detected and possibly removed.

For others, treatment may start with an exhortation to change their lifestyle, an approach that may well be strengthened with hypnosis.

If drug therapy is indicated, it escalates in complexity on a step-by-step basis.

Thiazide diuretics like bendrofluazide aim to reduce the volume of the blood.

Should these not have the desired result, the addition of a beta blocker, such as propranolol, can begin the process of reducing peripheral resistance.

The more recent drugs that have proved successful in this line are:

1. The *ACE* (angiotensin converting enzyme) *inhibitors.*
    Captopril was the original but there are now a whole market of variants blossoming behind it. They also lower peripheral resistance, easing the load on the heart.
2. Vasodilatation can be achieved by interfering with transport across cell membranes with the so-called *calcium antagonists.* Nifedipine is perhaps the best known.

It should not be forgotten that the aim of treatment is to produce the best possible distribution of blood at a pressure that is least damaging to the patient. Achieving this is clearly not easy. In the elderly, who may be well used to their level of blood pressure, exuberant reduction might well turn a simple ophthal-moscopic observation into a genuine disability.

In general terms the more pronounced the A/V crossing changes, the more likely treatment is to fail.

Once macular exudates have formed it is pointless to attempt their removal.

The ophthalmologist's role, however, is not just to confirm the findings made in a medical out-patient department:

1. the vision of eyes with central retinal vein occlusion can be saved to some degree
2. persistent vitreal haemorrhage can be cleared by vitrectomy

3.   the visual loss of arterial occlusion is usually irretrievable unless the block can be cleared within the hour.

Although the signs of hypertension can be detected in the eye, they are better discovered with the sphygmomanometer.

Hypertension behaves like chronic simple glaucoma. Patients do not know they have it until some vital organ has had it.

SUMMARY

The effects of rising blood pressure influenced by

1.   the state of the blood vessels
2.   rate of the pressure rise
3.   extent of pressure rise.

Young arterioles are wider with more elastic and muscles than those of later life, which fibrose into involutionary sclerosis. A/V crossing changes are the first real sign that hypertension is affecting the retina and possibly other parts of the body.

Dangers

1.   Macula — hard exudates in the form of a star can seriously damage central vision.
2.   Occlusion of the central retinal artery.
3.   Occlusion of the central retinal vein.

Hypertension is to the body what chronic simple glaucoma is to the eye. Both can exist unsuspected causing needless and irreversible destruction of special tissues.

15. Visual loss

THE REASONS WHY

By long tradition and common consent, chapters such as this have usually been entitled – 'Painless loss of vision'. There would then follow a procession of quite disconnected ocular disorders sharing only the absence of pain. Since this vast catalogue can be broken down into small groups and easily recognized by features which are present, it seems pointless to assemble a monstrous collection of conditions linked together only by one feature which is absent.

Vision can be lost for one of three reasons:

1. some disturbance of the clear media
   — the cornea
   — the aqueous
   — the lens
   — the vitreous

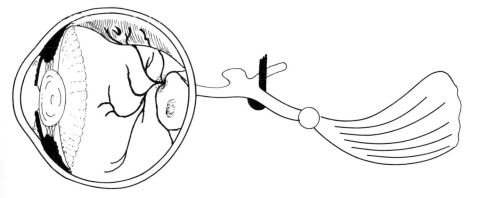

Fig. 15.1 Locating points of impairment of vision: 1) anterior to the chiasma – one eye; 2) at the chiasma – both sides; 3) posterior to the chiasma – one side.

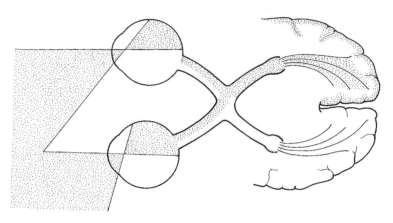

Fig. 15.2   The most common cause of homonymous hemianopia is blockage of the posterior cerebral artery. Blockage of the middle cerebral artery adds a hemiplegia as well.

2.   some disturbance in the retina
3.   some disturbance in the visual pathways
    — the optic nerve
    — the chiasma
    — post chiasmal pathways.

   In case we need reminding, the eye is an organ of limited response and what we must do is establish which area of the eye or visual pathways has been affected. Then and only then should we attempt to attach some explanatory pathological label to the defect.

   The following section deals with visual failure as perceived by the patient, using their own descriptions of companion symptoms and their time-scale. This means that some conditions will feature more than once because patients' perceptions of these conditions vary with their personality, their age and their general state of health.

Time-scale

Visual failure may be

1.   **transient** – returning to normal
2.   **sudden** – taking place over a second

3.   **rapid** – taking place over a week or so
4.   **indolent** – unremarkable in time to the patient.

Companion symptoms

We are now familiar with a range of what people complain about. Those relevant to visual failure are:

1.   no symptoms other than visual failure
2.   flickering and flashing lights
3.   floaters
4.   haloes
5.   a shadow in the visual field
6.   a shadow in the centre
7.   distortion
8.   diplopia.

TRANSIENT VISUAL LOSS

1.   **No companion symptoms** – patients complain of visual failure in one eye. Visual field contracts from the periphery inwards eventually clearing in the opposite direction.

Pathological basis

Vascular insufficiency in the internal carotid artery or its branches – ophthalmic artery backwards to the middle cerebral.

Clinical features

We generally learn of these from the patient's story otherwise the attack would not be transient.

The seven signs

No reason to reveal anything positive.

Fundus

No reason to be anything other than normal for the age group.

2. **Companion symptoms relating to the brain stem** –
    ataxia, vertigo, tinnitus, diplopia, nausea.

Pathological basis

Insufficiency of the vertebro-basilar arterial system.

The visual loss will tend to be homonymous, affecting the same visual field of each eye.

By the time we see the patient the episode will be past.

From the seven signs

No reason to be positive.

Fundus

Normal for the age group.

Action

These episodes must be regarded as serious evidence of possible impending stroke. The treatment is that of threatening cerebral thrombosis. Investigations must include:

1. an examination of the cardiovascular system including the great arteries to the head
2. a search for possible sources of ischaemia or relative ischaemia such as diabetes and the blood dyscrasias

Long term medication

Long term treatment with aspirin as an anticoagulant.

SUDDEN VISUAL LOSS

No companion symptoms

Total loss of light perception without warning in an elderly person means

1. central retinal artery occlusion
2. ischaemic optic neuropathy

Pathological basis

1. *Circulatory insufficiency* compounded by hypertension, diabetes and blood dyscrasias may be sufficient to block the central retinal artery.
2. *Inflammatory arteritis* – classically temporal arteritis is more common than might be thought and must be considered as the cause until proved otherwise.

1. Central retinal artery occlusion

From the seven signs
1. *Central vision*: total loss of light perception.
5. *Pupil*: no direct pupil response.

Fundus: An infarcted retina no longer transparent obscuring the choroid with its creamy whiteness everywhere except at the macula where it is too thin to prevent a view of the so-called cherry-red spot.

2. Ischaemic optic neuropathy

The seven signs are the same.
Fundus: a pale, swollen optic nerve head.

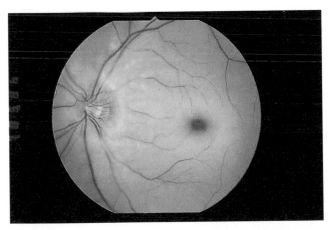

Fig. 15.3 Central retinal artery occlusion – the cherry-red spot, half remembered and never wholly understood. The macula dimples and hollows to its absolute centre where, even in its oedematous state, it allows the redness of the choroid to shine through when it is masked by oedema everywhere else.

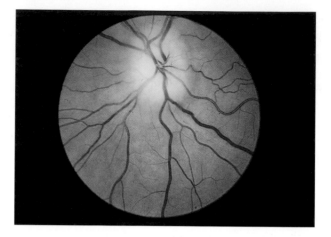

Fig. 15.4　Ischaemic optic neuropathy – a pale, swollen optic nerve head. Sudden loss of vision: think 'temporal arteritis'.

Action

1. *Central retinal artery occlusion*

The retina can survive ischaemia longer than can brain tissue and we have up to an hour to attempt to clear the blockage:

1.　vigorous massage of the globe can sometimes re-establish blood flow
2.　releasing fluid from the anterior chamber with a fine sharp blade (paracentesis) can sometimes soften the eye sufficiently to allow any thrombus or embolus to pass away from the main stem of the artery.

As might be guessed, success crowning such manoeuvres is more usually found in the original learned papers.

2. *Ischaemic optic neuropathy*

This condition and the previous one must be regarded as caused by temporal arteritis until a low ESR proves otherwise.

Systemic corticosteroids (e.g. prednisolone 50 mg daily) as a matter of some urgency. A temporal artery biopsy will then confirm the presence or absence of temporal arteritis. Although the passing euphoria induced by corticosteroids might tempt us to continue, if there is no evidence of arteritis they should be with-drawn before the catalogue of toxicity makes us wish they had been.

SUDDEN VISUAL LOSS

Companion symptoms: sudden gush of floaters – related to physical straining – elderly person

— vitreal haemorrhage.

Pathological basis

Bleeding – either spontaneous or in an eye vulnerable to such bleeding – diabetic, hypertensive.

From the seven signs

1. & 2.   *Central vision*: reduced.
3.   *Field vision*: intact

Fundus: black or swirling vitreal blood obscures red reflex.

Action

An ophthalmic surgeon in due course can determine if vitrectomy is indicated. Uncomplicated vitreal haemorrhage not infrequently will clear itself given time.

RAPID VISUAL LOSS

No companion symptoms:

— central retinal vein occlusion.

Pathological basis

— poor circulation
— diabetes
— hypertension
— blood dyscrasia
— chronic simple glaucoma.

From the seven signs

1. & 2.   *Central vision*: usually severely impaired.
5.   *Pupil*: poor direct light reflex (relative afferent pupillary defect compared with that of fellow eye).
7.   *Intraocular pressure*: raised if chronic simple glaucoma present.

The important thing is to detect any underlying systemic disorder. In the long term (3–4 months following the occlusion) there is the danger that ischaemic new blood vessel formation over the iris root may precipitate an acute rise in intraocular pressure in a very red eye.

An eye surgeon should be asked for an opinion – and of course urgently should acute pain develop.

RAPID VISUAL LOSS

Companion symptoms: flickering/flashing lights and floaters with a shadow in the peripheral vision

—   retinal detachment (see Fig. 10.8, p. 153).

Pathological basis

Vitreal traction on an abnormal patch of vitreal adhesion to the retina produces light flashing. As the retina gives way with the formation of a retinal tear, the retinal traction ends and so does the light flashing. Although it is classically stated that light flashing is synonymous with retinal detachment this is not the case. It occurs as described, during the formation of a retinal tear and when the tear has formed, it ceases.

The floaters result from pigment debris or frank haemorrhage being flung into the vitreal cavity.

The shadow relates directly to the area of lifting retina.

From the seven signs

1. & 2.   *Central vision*: reduced if macula involved.
3.   *Field vision* – a defect to hand movements will correspond to the area of the shadow.

Fundus: the view is characterized by a grey rippling reflex in place of the normal red reflex. The retina, transparent face on, becomes opaque in profile and obscures the underlying choroidal red glow together with the underlying choroidal detail.

Occasionally a vitreal haemorrhage prevents the appreciation of these subtleties.

SUDDEN VISUAL LOSS

Companion symptom: diplopia

— cranial nerve palsy, usually oculomotor.

Pathological basis

Diplopia usually dominates as a symptom because it is so gross but the oculomotor nerve also serves accommodation which will give rise to the appearance of visual loss.

Trauma or intracranial aneurysms of course take this out of the area of painless visual loss but diabetes brings it back within the limits of our remit.

From the seven signs

2. *Central vision* for *near*: diminished.
5. *Pupil*: dilated (usually).
   Cranial nerve examination will reveal ptosis and paralysis of all the eye movements except
      — downwards and inwards (4th nerve)
      — abduction (6th nerve).

Action

Even in the absence of pain one must assume an intracranial catastrophe until such is disproved.

Urgent referral for an ophthalmic opinion is indicated.

SUDDEN VISUAL LOSS

Companion symptoms: central shadow and distortion

— something at the macula.

   If macula intact, then

— something affecting the optic nerve or optic chiasma.

Something at the macula

Pathological basis

The macular region is extremely sensitive to damage:

1. *Haemorrhage* occurs in disciform degeneration of the elderly but may also occur in younger myopes.
2. *Background diabetic retinopathy* results in oedema, exudates and haemorrhages over the area of central vision.
3. *A branch of the central retinal vein* blocks for the same reasons as does the whole vein. Oedema in the central retina is what draws the patient's attention to the disorder.
4. *Central serous retinopathy.* This rare condition of young men usually results from a crack in one of the deeper ocular layers (Bruch's membrane) and collection of oedema in the sub-neuro-retinal space.
5. *Creeping retinal detachment.* It does happen from time to time that a retina, detaching because of a peripheral tear, may detach unnoticed until the macular retina separates also.

If fundal examination reveals none of these things at the macula then we have to think of the optic nerve itself.

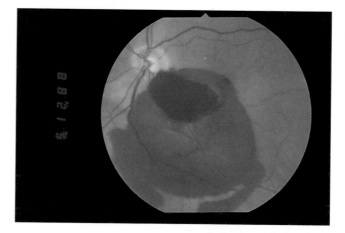

Fig. 15.5   Macular haemorrhage – usually the result of disciform degeneration, diagnosed here more from its position than its appearance, which is really that of another haemorrhage.

From the seven signs

1. & 2.   Common to all is loss of *central vision*.

Fundus: a haemorrhage at the macula is just that. It may take on various shapes, but the presence of blood dominates.

Diabetic macular changes will be seen as part of an overall background retinopathy.

A branch vein occlusion will be seen as a localised version of a total vein occlusion resulting in flame haemorrhages along the middle of the veins channelling above or below the macula back to the optic nerve head.

Central serous retinopathy

Fundus: to the unpractised eye the macula in this case may appear remarkably normal but we are looking for a 'blister' round the macular area.

Creeping retinal detachment

Fundus: The dominant feature will be the grey reflex that characterizes a detaching retina. The position cutting the macula will indicate why the patient has complained about it now.

Optic neuritis (retrobulbar neuritis)

Pathological basis

Demyelination usually hits one eye; viral neuritis may affect both.

A further **companion symptom** occasionally is pain on movement of the eye.

From the seven signs

1. & 2.   *Central vision*: diminished sometimes to light perception.
3   *Field vision*: may be normal, may be grossly restricted.
5   *Pupil*: poorly sustained light reflex.

Fundus: in optic neuritis the disc may be swollen. In retrobulbar neuritis the disc may be normal.

This is the condition where the patient sees nothing and the doctor sees nothing.

Action

Macula

Lesions at the macula are only urgent if something can be done about something. Once a macula has haemorrhaged enough to bring it to the patient's notice then it is probably too late.

Diabetic macular oedema, however, can be treated urgently with one of the new lasers. A branch retinal vein occlusion can also be treated in the same way.

Central serous retinopathy needs referral for diagnosis, upon which it is still possible that nothing may be done.

Retinal detachment the treatment of the macular problem is the treatment of the detachment.

The treatable conditions should be referred quickly because the quicker the macular lesion is attended to the better would be the central visual return.

Optic neuritis

If the neuritis is due to demyelination, as it usually is, then nothing will alter its course, usually to spontaneous recovery. It must be remembered that this could well be a harbinger of multiple sclerosis and it now has to be remembered also that the administration of systemic corticosteroids could hasten its recurrence.

Optic neuritis following a viral infection is usually bilateral and may well respond to systemic corticosteroids.

INDOLENT VISUAL LOSS

No companion symptoms:

— corneal opacity
— cataract
— chronic simple glaucoma
— secondary raised intraocular pressure (secondary glaucoma)
— retinal detachment
— central retinal vein occlusion
— intracranial compressive lesions (e.g. pituitary adenoma).

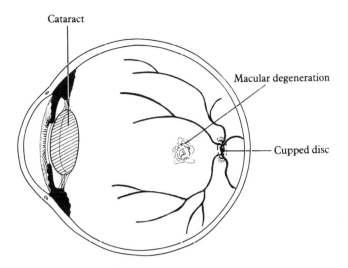

Cataract

Macular degeneration

Cupped disc

Fig. 15.6 Anyone old enough to have cataract or senile macular degeneration is old enough to have chronic simple glaucoma as well. 'Think aqueous.'

Pathological basis

The major long-term response of the cornea to insult is to lose its clarity – a response it shares with the lens. The precise insult does not matter. The response – loss of corneal transparency – does.

Keratoconus: the cornea of young astigmatic myopes can sometimes lose its regular curvature to become cone-shaped. Such coning increases the irregular astigmatism and destroys the cornea as an optical structure.

Cataract: surely the commonest cause of visual loss, particularly in the elderly. As with the cornea, the exciting insult is irrelevant, the response – a lens opacity – is not.

Chronic simple glaucoma: for a patient to recognize that something is wrong means that it has been permitted to go on for far longer than it should have.

Secondary rise in pressure: behaves in exactly the same way as chronic simple glaucoma and could very probably have been averted had the possibility been considered. The pressure mechanism, like so much else in the eye, has one response to insult – it ceases to work.

Retinal detachment: contrary to popular belief most retinal detachments do not flash with light but they can quietly destroy the vision in one eye whilst normality in its fellow gives the impression of normal vision.

Pituitary enlargement: although compression not affecting the macular fibres will damage only the visual field, the loss will not always be perceived as a shadow but simply as an overall blunting of vision.

Central retinal vein occlusion: whilst the thrombosis may happen over a short space of time, as with retinal detachment, its effects may be noticed only when the normal fellow eye is covered.

Cornea

From the seven signs

1. & 2.   *Central vision*: diminished.
4.   *Cornea*: opacity obvious to direct illumination and will be seen as an opacity against the red reflex with the pupil dilated.

Action

This is rarely an emergency and will respond in due course to corneal grafting if circumstances warrant it and if absence of pathological corneal new vessels permit it.

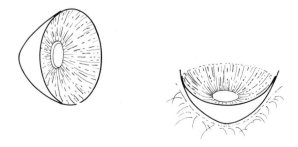

Fig. 15.7   Keratoconus – a moderately rare corneal dystrophy of early adult life. If a contact lens does not hold it in check, a corneal graft can clear the scar and the cone.

Keratoconus

From the seven signs

1. *Central vision,* particularly for *distance*: severely impaired and eventually uncorrectable with standard lens and eventually contact lenses.
4. *Cornea*: the coning can be seen in direct illumination when it has become pronounced. Looking downwards on the cornea from behind the patient allows the shape of the cone to be seen against the margin of the lower lid.

Action

Treatment is not straightforward.

Contact lenses were once thought to help prevent coning, although there is some evidence that they may increase it.

If progression appears inevitable then a corneal graft offers the best chance of visual return.

Cataract

Fundus

The opacities in the lens will be seen with the ophthalmoscope against the red reflex, and indeed may prevent any detailed view of the inside of the eye.

Action

Visual loss due to cataract is never urgent and removal is the only cure if cure be deemed necessary.

The age of cataract is also the age of chronic simple glaucoma and we should always think aqueous – has something happened to the aqueous flow? Is the pressure raised? Has 'glaucoma the process' started without our knowing it?

Chronic simple glaucoma (including secondary rise in intraocular pressure)

From the seven signs

3. *Field vision*: if unchecked, defects will be picked up on the nasal side of the hand movement field.

7. *Intraocular pressure*: raised (except in low-tension glaucoma where it appears normal).

Fundus: gross vertical cupping of the optic nerve head (see Fig. 12.4, p. 181).

Action

A high pressure and gross cupping call for fairly rapid referral, lest a central retinal vein occlusion destroy the remaining vision whilst the patient awaits a summons for ophthalmic examination.

Chronic glaucoma is a bilateral disease and we must always consider the other eye. A pressure rise secondary to some disorder will clearly damage only the affected eye.

Retinal detachment

From the seven signs

1. & 2.   *Central vision*: affected if the macula is involved.
3.   *Field vision*: loss corresponding to the symptomatic shadow.

Fundus: a grey rippling reflex.

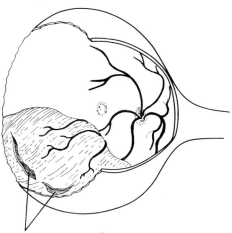

Break just behind ora serrata

Fig. 15.8   A creeping retinal detachment.

Action

If the macula is still attached, this is a matter of urgency. If the macula is already adrift, then referral need not take place on the day of discovery.

Intracranial compression (pituitary adenoma)

From the seven signs

1. & 2.   *Central vision*: loss relates to compression of the macular fibres at the chiasma.
3.   *Field vision*: bi-temporal field loss is classic and less rare.

Fundus: optic nerve head pallor.

Radiology, including CT scan, will demonstrate enlargement of the pituitary fossa.

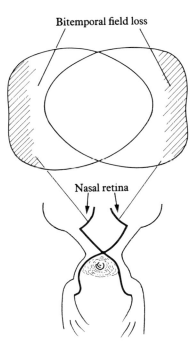

Fig. 15.9   Bitemporal field loss – can be detected with the hand movement field test.

Action

Referral to a neurosurgeon.

Central retinal vein occlusion

From the seven signs

1. & 2.   *Central vision*: usually greatly reduced but not always.
3.   *Field vision*: may be normal.
7.   *Intraocular pressure*: may be raised if venous occlusion is secondary to a hard eye.

Fundus: classic stormy sunset.

Action

Quiet referral for an ophthalmic opinion.

INDOLENT VISUAL LOSS

Companion symptoms: flickering, flashing floaters

— retinal detachment
— vitreal haemorrhage – plus retinal detachment
— vitreal haemorrhage – alone
— choroiditis.

Pathological basis

Flashing lights signify traction in the retina and they cease as soon as the traction has produced a retinal break.

Vitreal haemorrhage with or without retinal detachment

The tearing retina may include a blood vessel with an inevitable gush of blood into the vitreal cavity.

Vitreal haemorrhage does not always follow a retinal tear and may be caused by diabetes, hypertension or any of the bleeding disorders (including anticoagulant therapy).

Choroiditis

This is, happily, rare. Inflammation of the choroid can exude remarkable amounts of gelatinous material into the vitreal cavity.

Retinal detachment

The clinical features are the same as for any other detachment.

Retinal detachment plus vitreal haemorrhage

From the seven signs

3. *Field vision*: defects in the visual field may indicate that the loss is not uniform and will give the clue to a localized area of retinal elevation.

Fundus: vitreal blood may obscure details.

Action

Referral the next day allows the eye surgeon to determine, with ultrasound, if the retina is flat or not. If it is flat and no ongoing cause for bleeding remains untreated, then we may wait for the blood to clear. If it does not, we would proceed to vitrectomy.

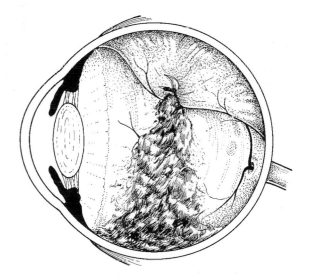

Fig. 15.10   Vitreal haemorrhage and retinal detachment.

Choroiditis

From the seven signs

1. & 2.   *Central vision*: blunted if the macula is involved.

Fundus: the red reflex dulled by vitreal haze.

Action

Referral over the next day or so.

INDOLENT VISUAL LOSS

Companion symptoms: a shadow in the peripheral field

— retinal detachment
— pituitary adenoma.

The pathological basis, clinical features and management have already been described.

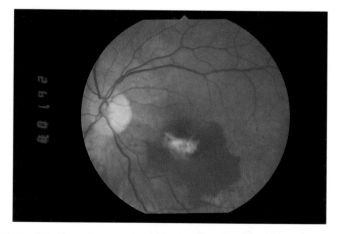

Fig. 15.11   Disciform degeneration of the macula. Macular change can take many forms. When bruised membrane cracks, new vessels forming from the choroid perforate into the sub-pigment-epithelial space, rupturing finally into the sub-neuro-retinal space with subsequent haemorrhage and scar formation and devastating effects on central vision.

INDOLENT VISUAL LOSS

Companion symptoms: shadow in the central area

— senile macular degeneration.

Pathological basis

Dry atrophy of the macula can take place over many years, quietly filing away at the central visual acuity.

From the seven signs

1. & 2.   *Central vision*: blunted.

Fundus: the macula will reveal:

1. atrophy
2. pigmentary disturbance
3. exudation
4. haemorrhage
5. scattered yellow dots.

   This is the age of chronic simple glaucoma and the patient may have this as well. Think aqueous!

Action

At the moment we have little to offer patients with dry macular degeneration. The condition often looks worse than it actually is and direct intervention with the laser can only make matters worse.

INDOLENT VISUAL LOSS

Companion symptoms: haloes and double vision

— cataract or corneal opacity.

Pathological basis

Interference with uniform clarity splits entering light into double images in one eye. It also results in a spectral break up, allowing a coloured ring to appear around lights. The haloes do not include all the colours of the spectrum but are usually variations on the orange theme. We must be sure that the diplopia is monocular.

From the seven signs

1. & 2.   *Central vision*: may be blunted.

Fundus: a cataract or, more rarely, corneal opacity will be seen against the red reflex.

People old enough to have cataract are old enough to have chronic simple glaucoma – think aqueous!

Action

Extraction of a cataract is not usually necessary when the major complaint is monocular double vision. Lens extraction is necessary only when complaints of double vision give way to complaints of major loss of vision.

SUMMARY

Fading vision can be frightening to both patient and doctor – to the former because of fears that worse is going to happen and to the latter because of uncomprehending terror of what has happened so far. The patient produces a string of apprehensive questions and the ophthalmoscope produces its customary blur.

Diagnoses will not cluster round the ophthalmoscope like moths just because we have switched on the light. They will, however, if we go through the seven signs first, using the ophthalmoscope as the eighth sign to confirm our suspicions, which after all is its primary role.

There is no need to contemplate the entire visual pathway and a comprehensive survey of its possible disorders with mounting horror. It splits quite distinctively into three sections, as do the possibilities. As to the disorders, they can be worked out from the roll-call of causation.

All we have to do is identify which part of the visual pathway is affected:

— cornea
— lens
— vitreous

— macular retina
— peripheral retina
— optic nerve back to occipital cortex.

The eye is an organ of limited response. And the segment of the eye responding can be easily identified once the seven signs have told us what we should be considering.

Anyone old enough to have one degenerative disorder is old enough to have the others, and the major three are:

1. cataract
2. chronic simple glaucoma
3. senile macular degeneration.

All three may exist in one eye.

Vascular accidents, because they are sudden, tend to attack one eye or one visual field at a time. Should the underlying condition be left unchecked, the other eye or field may follow rapidly.

Compression at the chiasma gives rise to defects in both visual fields – one lesion, both sides.

Lesions behind the chiasma affect the visual field of the other side – one lesion, one side.

Hypertension, as silent as chronic simple glaucoma, nibbles away unsuspected before showing its hand and trumping:

1. the eye with a venous or arterial occlusion – anterior to the chiasma therefore – one lesion, one eye
2. the brain with a stroke and the field with a homonymous hemianopia – behind the chiasma – therefore one lesion, one side.

The immediate effects of trauma are not painless; therefore they attract attention in their own right. The later effects, like secondary pressure rise and creeping retinal detachment, are frequently without symptoms and will only be caught in time if they are considered.

The answer to them all is not the ophthalmoscope. It is to go through the seven signs – alert to what might have happened, ready to change our mind if it appears that something else has happened and continually aware that, in the elderly, several things may have happened.

16. Painless swelling of the optic nerve head

A small cluster of disconnected conditions share the common sign of a swollen, or apparently swollen, optic nerve head. They divide into those which present:

1. with visual symptoms
2. without visual symptoms.

THOSE WITH VISUAL SYMPTOMS

Optic neuritis

This is one of those names which flash to mind from student days unaccompanied by any flash of enlightenment. Inflammation of the optic nerve head like inflammation anywhere else can develop as a result of local or remote infections but by far the highest proportion is due to demyelination. Most patients with optic neuritis will eventually go on to develop the general signs of multiple sclerosis.

Clinical features

The prime complaint is of visual loss and there may be a hint of pain on moving the eye.

The seven signs

1. & 2.   *Central vision – distance* and *near*: severely affected.
3.   *Field vision*: there is no single pattern, but the very extent makes it as dramatic and as obvious to the patient as loss in the centre.

5.   *Pupil*: response to light sluggish and poorly sustained. The accepted popular description is relative afferent pupil defect (RAPD).

Fundus

The optic nerve head

M — *Margin*: blurred
C — *Colour*: pink, or pinker than pink, or even red
C — *Cup*: reduced.

The retinal vessels could well be engorged.

There may be none of these fundal findings if the same process occurs further back along the optic nerve. It is at this point that optic neuritis is given the name of retrobulbar neuritis. The normally-appearing optic nerve head gives no hint of its presence. The other signs, of course, are the same. The patient sees nothing; the doctors sees nothing. It is just optic neuritis with its precise location further back in the nerve.

Ischaemic optic neuropathy

The elderly patient may develop acute anoxia of the optic nerve head – in both eyes. Should this occur we must assume a diagnosis of temporal arteritis until a temporal artery biopsy tells us that our suspicions were right or wrong.

A proportion of patients may develop all the symptoms and signs of this acute optic nerve head anoxia without any underlying arteritis.

Clinical features

The visual loss is painless, total and sudden in one eye and may be followed rapidly by the same in the other.

From the seven signs

1. & 2.   *Central vision* – distance and near – no light perception.
3.   *Field vision*: no light perception.
5.   *Pupil*: direct light reflex absent. Consensual reflexes present provided the fellow eye is normal when it is exposed to light.

Fundus

Optic nerve head

M — *Margin*: blurred
C — *Colour*: pale
C — *Cup*: obscured and filled with oedema.

We are dealing here with an ocular emergency. The second eye could follow suit with equal suddenness while the first eye is being pondered. A raised ESR indicates the need for systemic corticosteroids until an urgent temporal artery biopsy confirms or refutes the diagnosis.

Central retinal vein occlusion

Blockage of the central retinal vein produces, predictably enough, a flock of haemorrhages throughout the retina, together with oedema and swelling of the optic nerve head.

Clinical features

The first visual loss may be dramatic but its quiet occurrence may not be noticed since the blockage takes place over several hours or days and can well be ignored or totally missed.

From the seven signs

1. & 2.   *Central vision* – distance and near: may be severe but is never total. If ischaemia is limited there may be quite remarkable preservation of central vision.
5.   *Pupil*: direct light reflex sluggish. Consensual reflex normal provided the other eye is unaffected. An extreme and obvious relative afferent pupil defect is taken to indicate ischaemia.
7.   *Intraocular pressure*: may be raised and indeed may be the cause of the central retinal vein occlusion. To complicate the matter further, however, it may also be totally normal. A faltering blood flow can be tipped into frank stasis by chronic elevation of the intraocular pressure. The most common cause of this elevation is chronic simple glaucoma.

THOSE WITHOUT VISUAL SYMPTOMS

Papilloedema

A choked optic nerve head is the classic sign of raised intracranial pressure. In itself it has no immediate effect on vision and patients will present with symptoms and signs quite remote from the eye. Indeed they may present with neither.

The actual cause remains unexplained. It is, however, generally agreed that elevation of the levels of cerebrospinal fluid transmitted along the sheaths of the optic nerves is an initiating factor.

Thereafter, as a secondary phenomenon, the venous drainage from the eye becomes blocked and, more subtly still, there is some disturbance in an axoplasmic transport, resulting in white debris on the optic nerve head and within its microcirculation.

This usually bilateral appearance must be taken as a sign of raised intracranial pressure. There are causes other than a cerebral tumour. Papilloedema is the sign that changes severe hypertension into malignant hypertension.

Benign intracranial hypertension – a condition sometimes associated with the contraceptive pill – gives rise to optic nerve head

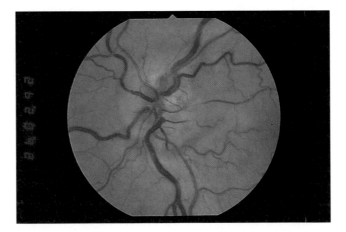

Fig. 16.1   Papilloedema – a swollen optic nerve head – characterised by loss of clarity of the disc margins and engorgement of the retinal veins. If due to papillitis, vision may be extinguished. If due to simple mechanical back pressure, vision may be unaffected.

swellings quite as spectacular as those associated with any other more serious lesion.

Clinical features

There are no symptoms referable to the papilloedema but there may be symptoms referable to the cause of the papilloedema. Tumour symptoms – headache is usually of recent origin and of progressive intensity. Not all intracranial tumours present with headache, however.

From the seven signs

There may be nothing positive.

Fundus

The optic nerve head

M — *Margin*: blurred and concealed
C — *Colour*: florid
C — *Cup*: obliterated by the oedema of the engorged optic nerve head.

The retinal veins may be swollen and a few local haemorrhages complete the picture. They are never as dramatic as those of venous occlusion, where the visual loss makes the distinction unmistakable.

Papilloedema is usually discovered incidentally. But if we have gone about things in order, it should be the last finding in the ophthalmic sequence. We may well have picked up a field defect or a curious pupil on the way.

The history can then be extended and a cranial nerve assessment is as far as an ophthalmologist is usually competent to take the clinical examination.

If malignant hypertension is discovered at this point then it has really been discovered too late. It should be found in the arm with a sphygmomanometer.

Investigation of intracranial disease has been greatly simplified by the introduction of the CT scan (computerised tomography). It may well reach a diagnostic conclusion on an out-patient basis without the infernal apparatus which used to preface surgery on the brain.

Pseudopapilloedema

Apparent swelling of the optic nerve head can mimic superficially the appearances of genuine swelling and the distinction is not always so clear-cut that we can sleep easily on a clinical impression.

1. The small, crowded eyes of long sight and astigmatism have small, crowded discs where there is not enough room for all the normal structures to spread out.
2. Drusen – deposition of hyaline material in the optic nerve head – can obliterate the cup and blur the margins and cause considerable diagnostic effort to someone unlucky enough to pick up the appearance as an incidental finding.

Clinical features

There are no clinical features referable to pseudopapilloedema but gross long sight and astigmatism will have produced at least a history of visits to an optician and of glasses prescribed, worn or abandoned.

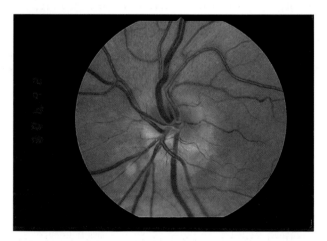

Fig. 16.2   Pseudopapilloedema. The distinction from genuine papilloedema cannot be made by the absence of symptoms. Normal veins, normal cranial nerves and long sight all point to pseudopapilloedema. If they do not point with sufficient lack of ambiguity, an intravenous fluorescein angiogram would prove the case beyond doubt.

From the seven signs

1. *Central vision – distance*: the long-sighted eye may require help in the distance with a pin hole.
2. *Central vision – near*: the long-sighted eye uses up its reading focus to see in the distance, and even in young patients there may be difficulty with near vision.
6. *Anterior chamber*: may be shallow – the long-sighted eye is small in every way.
7. *Intraocular pressure*: no reason to be raised unless a hypermetropic eye is edging towards acute angle closure.

Fundus

Optic nerve head

M — *Margin*: it is the blurred edges that attract attention
C — *Colour*: the dark redness gives the impression of swelling
C — *Cup*: may well be obliterated.

There will also be no symptoms, but there will be greater anxiety, when this chance finding has been made.

Should any doubt exist, it is possible to dispel it with an intravenous fluorescein angiogram. Sodium fluorescein injected into one of the arm veins can be traced as it flows through the eye, demonstrating by its normal passage or by leakage the absence or presence of an abnormal swelling of the optic nerve head.

Drusen, when exposed to blue light, fluoresce even without the injection of sodium fluorescein, giving away the diagnosis immediately.

SUMMARY

Oedema of the optic nerve head can develop in:

1. *papillitis* – optic neuritis of the optic nerve head, usually due to demyelination
2. *vascular* – ischaemic optic neuropathy – temporal arteritis assumed and confirmed by a raised ESR and artery biopsy. Central retinal vein occlusion, chronic simple glaucoma, diabetes, hypertension must all be considered and looked for
3. *papilloedema* – raised intracranial pressure must be assumed but CT scans have reduced the misery of preoperative investigation

4. *pseudopapilloedema* – the appearance of a swollen optic nerve
   head, either the result of a small, long-sighted eye or of
   hyaline deposits.

17. AIDS

Although a lively controversy has been sparked off by the allegation that the human immunodeficiency virus (HIV) does not obey Koch's postulates, this retrovirus is generally accepted as the cause of the acquired immunodeficiency syndrome in humans which we call AIDS.

The condition has been recognized in sub-Saharan Africa for over 40 years where its capacity to shrink victims to almost skeletal levels has acquired for it the popular name of 'slim'.

Its entry to Europe and the Western world cannot be exactly dated. The first known case was probably in the early sixties although it was not diagnosed at the time. An English soldier died of a wasting condition that baffled his medical attendants. Doubtless they went through the correct examination procedures and, against the knowledge available at the time, they drew a blank.

It might be worth a mention that the existence of diseases not yet described must be the final argument against the syndrome approach to diagnosis, still so popular amongst ophthalmologists, whereby the examination sequence alters to fit the supposed condition, merely confirming by rote what we already know by instinct. This system collapses completely when we do not know in advance what is wrong and thus can have no way of knowing which collection of signs to use in anticipation.

The physicians in charge of the soldier had the foresight to retain some of his serum, which has since tested positive for HIV.

TRANSMISSION

There are two prime modes of infection and both involve entry of the virus into the circulation either by:

1. *parenteral intravenous injection* – common in drug abusers and unhappily discovered in haemophiliacs transfused with infected blood
2. *intimate sexual contact* – originally limited to homosexuals but now all contacts, irrespective of sex, and finally, the most tragic of all, babies of infected mothers, without choice, who begin their lives HIV-positive.

And on into the complaisant world of sex for money, where we should not forget package holidaymakers lured by an Apex fare on a plane to a fanfare of strumpets somewhere else. They either do not know or do not care but, having acquired their infection at a discount, they spread it about for nothing.

The full impact of AIDS on all our societies has yet to be felt. In Africa and the Far East the predicted infection rates and the inevitable impact on the social fabric of the countries involved are both unimaginable and fearful.

PATHOGENESIS

Upon initial infection, the virus attaches to and enters target cells in the host, which mainly comprise T-helper lymphocytes, monocytes and macrophages. In these cells viral RNA is transcribed into single-stranded RNA by the action of an enzyme – reverse transcriptase.

The viral genome integrates with the host chromosome and may remain quiescent, latent and unsuspected for years. The carriers look just like anyone else and even they may not realise that some random, long-forgotten encounter has turned them into someone dangerous to know. This dark menace haunting the next generation casts a shadow today like that of syphilis a century ago.

Reactivation of the latent infection may occur in time, leading to a loss of host-cell-mediated immunity. The patient will suffer infections off and on for no apparent reason. And, like syphilis, the infecting organism may target specific organs such as the central nervous system.

CLINICAL FEATURES

Most people will be unaware that they have acquired any infection unless they suspect they have been in circumstances where it was possible. Some, however, develop an acute brief febrile illness not unlike infectious mononucleosis within 3–6 weeks of exposure.

Antibodies to HIV do not begin to develop in any recognizable way until at least a month following transmission and in many cases the latent period may be as long as 3 months. Eventually, after long asymptomatic periods, most infected patients develop

a generalized lymphadenopathy
— weight-loss and malaise
— infections such as *Candida* or herpes zoster
— persistent disturbance of blood constituents.

All these apparent chance happenings may be heralds of the full-blown syndrome of AIDS, with profound cellular immuno-deficiency leading to opportunistic infections, tumours, dementia and death.

There is still some debate about which people are unlucky enough to develop the full-blown syndrome. A study has revealed that after $7^{1}/_{2}$ years, 30% of all patients known to be sero-positive have developed AIDS, the onset of which may be delayed by Zidovudine.

OPPORTUNISTIC INFECTIONS

Inevitably the reduced resistance to casual pathogens opens the door to random infection by:

1. *Pneumocystis carinii*
2. *Toxoplasma*
3. *Candida*
4. *Cryptococcus*
5. *Microbacterium*
6. cytomegalovirus
7. herpes simplex virus
8. herpes zoster virus

Pneumonia must be the most common incidental condition in this group.

Direct replication of the virus within the mononuclear cells of the central nervous system can result in progressive dementia which can affect up to half of all people with AIDS. The meninges, the brain itself, and indeed peripheral nerves as well, may all succumb to casual infection.

Certain malignancies would appear to be more common, such as Kaposi's sarcoma and various types of lymphoma.

OCULAR COMPLICATIONS

Like syphilis, AIDS is the great simulator – attacking aggressively without apparent restraint any bodily system.

Retinal vascular disease

Asymptomatic transient disturbances of the retinal microvascular circulation commonly occur. The retinal changes are not pathognomonic of AIDS; they are merely pathognomonic of retinal changes that occur in response to circulatory disturbance whatever the cause.

This is in line with the eye's standard behaviour of having a limited response, indeed almost the same response, to a multiplicity of different agencies. The changes described here are faintly reminiscent of those found in diabetic retinopathy, and in a sense follow the same pattern, but clearly the exciting reason is different. The capillaries, being incompetent, may

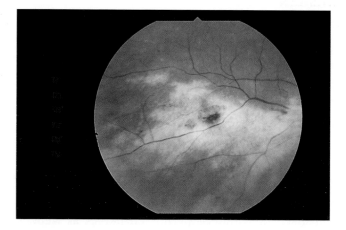

Fig. 17.1 CMV retinitis. The cream and ketchup appearance – a prelude to retinal necrosis.

1. bulge in small areas – producing microaneurysms
2. bulge over extended areas – producing intraretinal microvascular abnormalities (IRMA)
3. leak – producing retinal haemorrhages
4. block the passage of blood – producing cotton-wool spots (ischaemia).

Ocular infections

1. Herpes zoster ophthalmicus (shingles) differs only because of its increased severity.
2. Herpes simplex produces dendritic ulcers in the cornea in those who are immuno-incompetent.
3. CMV retinopathy – almost half of AIDS patients suffer this infection of the retina at some stage of their disease. It is characterized by yellow-white patches that obscure the choroid outside the vascular arcades. The development of haemorrhage within and at the edges of these lesions has provoked the ghastly description of 'cheese and ketchup', which could only have come from the land of the burger bar – where the container is often tastier than the contents.

    In time these patches become atrophic. The retinal necrosis and perforations finally result in detachment of the retina.

MANAGEMENT

As can be guessed, in the face of this appalling destruction of the body's defences we have little to offer on a long-term basis. An antiviral DNA analogue – ganciclovir, similar to acyclovir – can, if injected intravenously, halt progression of the lesions. The virus, however, is not eradicated and the retinopathy occurs as soon as treatment is stopped. As can be guessed, the treatment itself is not without its own form of morbidity.

18. The cerebral connection

Headaches and the cranial nerves

In the ophthalmic out-patient clinic, there is neither time nor space to do justice to a full neurological examination. In any case there is rarely any point, because neurologists do it better and, if we have been moved to consider it ourselves, we have probably suspected something that is going to require the services of a neurologist anyway.

As ophthalmologists, however, we are regularly faced with a variety of complaints that have more than a hint of a neurological component and we are not infrequently the final despairing port of call for patients with headaches that can apparently be neither diagnosed or treated.

HEADACHE

Patients with pain in the head come our way for three main reasons:

1. they may have pain in or about the eye
2. they may have pain anywhere in the head together with visual symptoms such as flashing lights
3. we may be the last despairing hope of a referring doctor in search of an ocular explanation for headaches that have defied every other attempt at explanation.

Pain in the eye

This section might reasonably start with a couplet that owes more of its rhyme, elegance and rhythm to the Bard of the Tay, William McGonagall, than to Alexander Pope:

If pain in the eye is caused by the eye,
We don't have to look for the reason why.

For those who require a prosaic interpretation of the preceding poetry, ocular causes of ocular pain are obvious – often without any need for the seven signs.

A red eye is unmistakable because it is a red eye which happens to have produced a headache.

Only very occasionally are apparently quiet eyes to blame, and in such cases a diagnosis can be achieved from the history.

If there is some binocular imbalance producing discomfort in the use of the eyes, then the patient will tell us so.

Binocular abnormalities

Uncorrected refractive errors, extremely dry eyes etc. will produce discomfort on use which clears when the eyes are rested or shut.

Headache plus visual symptoms

For all practical purposes the symptoms are almost always flashing lights which, in the absence of a convincing story of migraine, are feared to be an indication of some underlying potential ocular disaster.

Idiopathic migraine usually begins in adolescence. There may be a family history of this tendency – on questioning, troubled adults may also remember episodes of travel sickness in their childhood.

There are all manner of triggers but most patients are usually aware that something is going to happen. They may experience sensations of listless ill-temper and intolerance of assaults on their special senses of eyes, ears and nose. It is at this time that the visual sensations develop. The vision itself may diminish or may be augmented by bright lights flickering in the temporal field. There may even be a field defect. These symptoms are generally explained by arterial constriction and by ischaemia of either the retina or brain or both.

When the aura passes and function returns, the headache commences – usually unilateral and not infrequently beside or behind the eye.

This phase is thought to be due to dilating blood vessels which stretch the main fibres in the vessel walls.

Cluster headaches

A series of these headaches, usually over a period of weeks, concentrate in one eye of the middle-aged. They may occur every night, breaking sleep and marked by swelling and tenderness in the adjacent skin.

Headaches without explanation

Although the word migraine is bandied about with great fluency, most headaches are caused by something else, though that is not to say what causes them can be readily identified. Most headaches in fact are not caused by any underlying disease. Transient causes like too much whisky or gross self-indulgence of one sort or another are easily recognized.

For those unlucky enough to suffer persistent headaches with no preceding entertainment, the assumption that it must indicate something sinister is perfectly sensible. The irony is that this assumption is almost always wrong.

Headaches which come and go and perhaps come more often than they go over a period of months are usually the result of stress or tension or anxiety or depression. They are not associated with any generalized symptoms suggestive of serious intracranial disease.

The brain is housed in a cavity with rigid walls. If any lesion within this cavity occupies space that does not belong to it, then it may certainly produce headache but this will be of recent onset, usually unremitting and also associated with other evidence of disturbed cerebral function.

The higher centres will respond with fluctuating consciousness and indeed fluctuating comprehension.

The special senses or any of the cranial nerves may be involved to some degree.

Interference with motor or sensory innervation will be identified as muscle weakness or as numbness.

Acute headaches with an obvious underlying cause such as inflammation or infection of adjacent structures such as:

1. the meninges
2. the sinuses
3. the teeth

4.   the ears
5.   the temporal arteries

should usually be obvious because they are in reality headaches plus something else.

Temporal arteritis is particularly sinister because the something else may turn out to be ischaemic optic neuropathy – a total loss of vision in one or both eyes which might have been averted had the cause of the headache been considered to begin with.

Serious intracranial disease

When we as ophthalmologists are faced with symptoms which appear to stem from the central nervous system we can, to begin with, avoid the need for neurological assistance by carrying out two simple sets of investigations:

1.   an assessment of the cranial nerves
2.   radiography of the skull.

THE CRANIAL NERVES

The most serious flaw in what should be a simple clinical sequence is that we tend to feel clinically insecure as we move into the

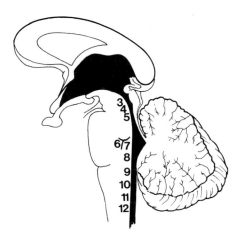

Fig. 18.1   Although certain cranial nerve nuclei are companions in the brain stem, the nerves themselves may separate. The approximate brain-stem levels of the nuclei can give useful locating information.

higher centres above the brain stem. There may well be two reasons for such an uneven grasp. To begin with, the tests for the optic nerve are generally taught by a physician, who doubtless learnt them from another physician who probably delighted in spot diagnosis with the ophthalmoscope.

Probably of much greater consequence is something altogether more ridiculous. It would appear to be the universal experience of us all that somewhere between the seventh and eighth cranial nerve, brains cloud over with hunger and the mysterious secrets of the remaining four disappear forever with the teacher to the dining room.

The following section will give equal weight to all the nerves.

Olfactory

Although officially called a nerve, this is anatomically part of the brain. In theory, each nostril – free of phlegm – should be offered some familiar non-irritant volatile oil, like wintergreen or oil of cloves. Sadly, when we look for them, we tend to find in practice that the oils have been abducted, possibly for some humble therapeutic reason. It is therefore customary to bypass the first nerve, with perhaps a question or two about the sense of smell.

Optic nerve

Like the olfactory nerve, this is strictly brain tissue. It serves two different functions:

1. it conducts impulses of vision from the retina to the visual cortex.
2. it is the inflow arm of the pupil reflexes carrying certainly information about illumination, though less certainly about accommodation to the mid brain, where the sign tuning of pupil size is selected before passing through the ocular motor nerve to the pupil.

These two aspects of function are tested routinely.

1. The three visions:
    a. *central – distance* and *near*
    b. *field*
    At this point in a textbook of ophthalmology they cannot need to be discussed further.

2. The *pupil* – light and accommodation. Briskness of response and equality and size are the two prime features that indicate normal pupils.

Since we always run the risk of being asked for our views on this or that pupil anomaly it would seem sensible now to consider some of them – both pathological and physiological.

The Argyll Robertson pupil

A famous defect associated with cerebral syphilis, this is recognized by a small irregular pupil that fails to respond to the strongest light. However it does respond to near focus. The old mnemonic was to compare it with student lodgings of a former generation, as having accommodation but no light.

The Holmes-Adie pupil

This myotonic pupil, not associated with cerebral syphilis, is rather larger than normal and, although not responding promptly

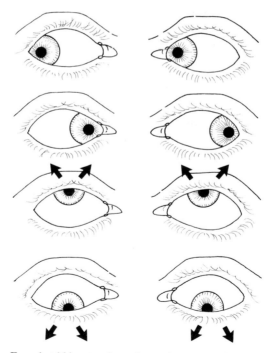

Fig. 18.2 Eyes should be tested together and separately. It is particularly important to push the movements to the limits of gaze.

to light and accommodation, will do so eventually, given enough time, and will take as long again to relax.

Associated with loss of focus and also with loss of tendon reflexes, it is perhaps more common in young women.

Constriction of such a pupil by mecholyl – a parasympathetic agent – in concentrations that would have no effect on a normal pupil passes from textbook to textbook as a mandatory element of diagnosis. It is generally in the textbook that it remains, for by the time the unstable solution has been prised from the grasp of a reluctant pharmacist, its potency will have gone, and indeed so may have the patient.

Pilocarpine weakened to 0.1% is just as effective and infinitely more stable. That it is so does not greatly matter, for clinical diagnosis is usually enough.

Horner's syndrome

A small pupil and a dropped eyelid (ptosis), together with mild sinking of the globe into the orbit (enophthalmos), make up a popular exam question.

The pathological basis lies in paralysis of the cervical sympathetic nervous system, and possible causes can be found in the standard catalogue of disease causation.

Clearly trauma, neoplasia and inflammation etc. can catch the sympathetic fibres around the great vessels at the root of the neck, and a bronchogenic carcinoma at the apex of the lung is an answer that the examiners are frequently looking for, coupled with homilies on the evils of tobacco.

Traumatic mydriasis

A blow on the eye may paralyse the pupil sphincter. A penetrating injury of the eye can actually prolapse part of the pupil through the wound.

Other distortions can be worked out from the common list of causation.

Trauma to the head has two distinct effects:

— in the early phases where irritation dominates, the pupil tends to constrict
— in later stages when the intracranial pressure is rising, dilatation of the pupil would confirm that the phase of irritation has given way to the phase of compression.

Drugs

Any sympathomimetic agent will dilate the pupil, as will alcohol.
Constriction is brought about parasympathomimetic agents, and of course the pin-point pupils of heroin addiction are unmistakable.

Oculomotor, trochlear and abducent

Though not strictly chronological, it makes sense to take the third, fourth and sixth cranial nerves together, because the structures they innervate also work together.

Oculomotor

The third nerve controls three different functions:

1. its parasympathetic fibres form the outflow for reflex control of the pupil
2. part of its motor fibres supply the levator muscle of the upper lid
3. its other motor fibres innervate the movement of the eye in all directions except those innervated by the fourth and sixth nerves.

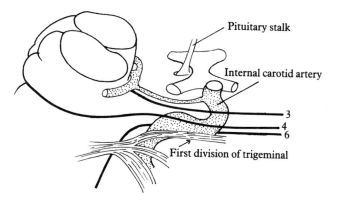

Fig. 18.3   Misadventures around the pituitary fossa can involve many structures. The optic nerves are vulnerable to aneurysm. The optic chiasma can be compressed by a swelling pituitary gland. Involvement of the third, fourth, fifth and sixth nerves implicates the cavernous sinus rather than the brain stem.

Trochlear

If the eye cannot be adducted (third nerve palsy) then an intact superior oblique will not be able to rotate the eye downwards with any great conviction. However, when the superior oblique comes into action in an unsuccessful attempt at downward movement it will produce rotation instead. The rotation is on an axis running through the pupil to the optic nerve and the superior oblique is at its most active as an internal rotator of the eye (intorsion) when the eye is abducted.

If some pigmentary fleck in the iris (there is always one somewhere) can be identified, then its rotation on the pupillary axis indicates a functioning trochlear nerve.

Abducent

The sixth cranial nerve innervates the lateral rectus.

Tests

It is customary to examine the movements of each eye separately. Monocular movements are known as ductions.

Binocular movements are known as versions.

1. pupil light reflex (see p. 64)
2. levator action – is there ptosis?
3. extraocular ductions (one eye at a time)

It is critical to push each movement to its limit (p. 260). A third nerve palsy will result in

1. a dilated pupil
2. a dropped upper lid (ptosis)

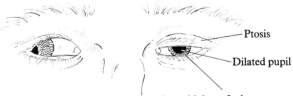

Ptosis

Dilated pupil

Failure of adduction together with loss of other movements

Fig. 18.4   A third nerve palsy is marked by ptosis, a dilated pupil and loss of all movements except abduction and intorsion. To note whether the pupil is spared or not is a nicety, for the cause is still an aneurysm unless investigation proves the assumption wrong.

3. paralysis of all eye movements except that of
    a. superior oblique (nerve 4) – intorsion
    b. lateral rectus (nerve 6) – abduction

Superior oblique: An isolated palsy of this muscle is rare.
Test: The order to 'look down' is not followed by any downward movement of the adducted eye.
Abducent: An isolated palsy of this muscle is common.
Test: Limitation of abduction – end-point nystagmus

Trigeminal

This fifth cranial nerve is the main sensory innervator of the face, in three great branches:

1. ophthalmic
2. maxillary
3. mandibular.

Its distribution spreads from the forehead and temples to the lower jaw.

We are of course particularly interested in its ophthalmic branch, which supplies pain sensation to the eye. Less obvious structures supplied by this nerve include the sinuses, all the contents of the mouth and the hard palate.

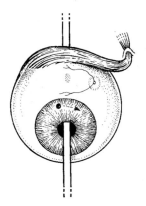

Fig. 18.5 The superior oblique (trochlear nerve) depresses the eye in adduction. If the eye cannot adduct, the superior oblique cannot depress the eye. When it tries to, it produces intorsion instead.

The soft palate and the posterior third of the tongue belong to nerves nine and ten (glossopharyngeal and vagus). The motor element of this nerve supplies the muscles of mastication.

Test

1. Compare the right and left sensation to touch along areas supplied by the three divisions:
    — temple
    — cheeks
    — chin.
2. Feel the masseters when the teeth are clenched.

Facial

The seventh nerve is mainly motor to the muscles of facial expression. However, it also carries:

1. parasympathetic secretory fibres to the lacrimal gland
2. taste fibres to the anterior two-thirds of the tongue.

Tests

Motor: In the event of a seventh nerve palsy, the normal fellow muscle pulls the paralysed muscle towards the normal side.

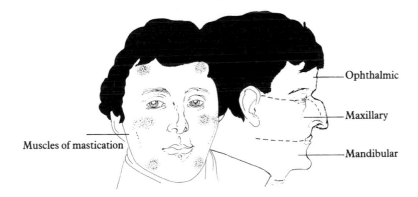

Fig. 18.6 Sensations on the temple, cheek and chin, as well as the cornea and buccal mucous membranes, are served by the three great divisions of the trigeminal nerve. The muscles of mastication are served by the motor root.

Blowing out the cheeks sometimes exposes a minimal weakness. Requests to whistle and smile are more likely to produce embarrassment than information.

The muscles of the forehead have bilateral representation in the motor cortex. This fact allows us to decide whether a palsy of the seventh nerve is due to the nerve itself or to some derangement of the higher connections.

In a lower motor neurone palsy, the fact that the nerve has bilateral cortical representation is irrelevant because the normal impulses cannot be passed along the damaged nerve. For that reason the entire side of the face, including the forehead, will be immobile, unwrinkled and expressionless.

In an upper motor neurone palsy the whole forehead (upper part of the face) will continue to wrinkle in the normal way. Only the lower part of the face will be dragged towards the normal side.

Sensory: Tradition demands that we test the sensation in the anterior two thirds of the tongue for

1. sweet (sugar)
2. sour (citric acid)
3. bitter (quinine)
4. salt (obvious).

Tradition does not always, however, have its demands met because, as with the volatile oils, the necessary materials have

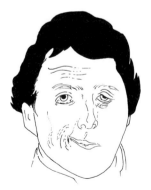

Fig. 18.7 The forehead is spared when an upper motor neuron lesion paralyses the seventh cranial nerve, but not when the nerve itself is damaged. The healthy side pulls the weakened side towards it. Theory calls for examination of the taste in the anterior two thirds of the tongue – a call not always needed.

generally vanished or their labels have. To search for them is rarely worth the effort.

Acoustic

The eighth nerve serves both hearing and balance.

Hearing

Tests: The auditory component can be checked by presenting an unobtrusive noise to each ear. The forefinger fretting against the thumb requires no equipment. The inclusion of quartz movements into Swiss timepieces has now made watches that tick almost antique. Whispering, which might appear fun to some patients, could well appear suggestive to others.

Needless to say the triumphant discovery of deafness could well mean an earful of wax.

If genuine deafness is discovered, we may proceed to the tuning fork, if that has not disappeared along with the citric acid, the quinine and the volatile oils.

The names Rinne and Weber may well have been the last pearls cast before teaching of the cranial nerves came to a halt. The result is that most people remember the names but rarely their significance.

The conduction of noise through air is more efficient than through bone, provided the middle ear is intact. A vibrating fork

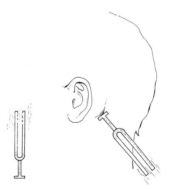

Fig. 18.8   The finger and thumb rubbed together in the well-known 'money' gesture can be heard by the average ear. Tuning forks can also be heard, but cannot always be found.

is placed on the mastoid until it is heard no more (bone conduction). Then it is placed by the open ear (air conduction).

1. The normal ear will hear it – because air conduction is better than bone conduction.
2. The ear with middle ear disease will not hear it (bone conduction better than air conduction because the middle ear is diseased).
3. The ear with nerve deafness will not hear it at all – either through bone or air. Conduction is irrelevant if there is no central nerve to pick it up.

Balance

Tests: Changing position of the head in space is reflected in fluid movements within the semicircular canals. If the head be held static and the semicircular canals can be stimulated, then eyes can be induced to move provided the vestibular apparatus is normal.

Stimulation of the semicircular canals can be induced by changing the temperature adjacent to them. The simplest way to achieve this is to pour hot or cold water into the external ear. A resultant nystagmus will twitch one way for hot – the other way for cold.

Pouring water into the external ear may be simple but it is by no means pleasant. It is also quite upsetting. It is perhaps wiser to leave the neurologists not only to interpret the subtle findings but also to parry the more vociferous complaints that sometimes appear to be the main response to this intrusion.

Glossopharyngeal

The ninth cranial nerve innervates movements of the soft palate and supplies sensation to the pharynx and its neighbours, together with a sense of taste for the posterior third of the tongue.

Tests

When the patient says 'aah', the pharynx:

1. in health constricts, raising the uvula in the central line
2. in disease constricts only on the healthy side, moving the uvula to that side.

Paralysed side

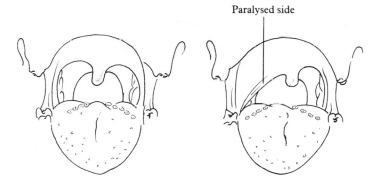

Fig. 18.9   To ask the patient to say 'aah' is not to place the doctor in a position of superiority. It arches the healthy palate and fails to arch the side supplied by a non-functioning glossopharyngeal nerve and vagus nerve. As with a seventh nerve palsy, the weak side is dragged towards the healthy side.

This behaviour is very like that of the facial nerve on the normal side in a seventh nerve palsy.

The gag reflex induced by touching the pharynx will for some of us bring back recollections of jolly evenings or of less jolly examinations by an ear, nose and throat surgeon. It probably produces little except declining cooperation by the time we come to the tenth, eleventh and twelfth nerves.

Anyone who has tried even to see the posterior third of the tongue will quickly realize that it is asking too much of patients to distinguish between sweet, sour, bitter and salt while they are trying hard not to vomit.

Vagus

The tenth cranial nerve plays many roles, but in essence:

1.   it joins the ninth in the movements of the soft palate
2.   it innervates the extrinsic muscles of the larynx
3.   it slows the heart
4.   it excites secretion and movement of the gut.

Tests

Even the abbreviated function seems formidable to test. In reality, watching the soft palate and the uvula with the ninth is all that we

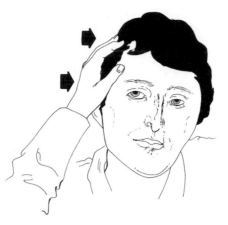

Fig. 18.10   The accessory nerve innervates the head turn and shoulder shrug.

require. Other malfunctions – changes in the voice or dysphagia – rapidly indicate that the ophthalmologist should withdraw both gracefully and gratefully.

Accessory

The eleventh cranial nerve is involved with the tenth, as the tenth is with the ninth, but its main role is to innervate the trapezius and the sternomastoid muscles.

Tests

Shoulder shrugging and rotating the head against resistance tell us all we need to know.

Hypoglossal

The random connections of the twelfth cranial nerve are as nothing compared with its motor supply to the tongue.

The normal tongue emerges straight – a movement not encouraged in most cultures.

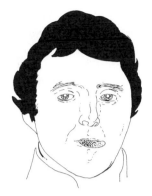

Fig. 18.11   With a hypoglossal palsy, the tongue is pushed towards the damaged side. This is in direct contrast to facial palsy and palatal palsy when the face and the palate are pulled towards the normal side.

Test

Should the tongue be paralysed on one side, it cannot actively protrude on that side. The healthy muscle, on the other hand, can and does protrude and pushes the tongue to the weakened side. This shift to the paralysed side is quite opposite to what happens in the case of a facial or glossopharyngeal palsy, when the shift is to the healthy side.

RADIOGRAPHY OF THE SKULL

In certain cases a radiograph of the skull – as the limit of our investigation – might give information on the following points:

1. The pituitary fossa – a large fossa indicates a large gland, and a large gland can compress the visual pathways into field defects and optic atrophy, which may mimic those of chronic glaucoma.
2. Abnormal calcification sometimes outlines the wall of a carotid aneurysm or disperses within the substance of a tumour.
3. Disturbance of intra-cranial bone, like hyperostosis, could well indicate a meningioma or some less common growth.

SUMMARY

Persistent recurrent headaches with no companion symptoms rarely indicate serious intracranial disease.

Headaches of recent identifiable onset, if a symptom of serious intracranial disease, will usually be part of a symptom complex involving either:

1. the higher cerebral functions
2. state of consciousness
3. the special senses
4. the cranial nerves
5. peripheral motor and sensory distribution.

19. Nystagmus

Nystagmus may be defined as an involuntary repetitive oscillation of one or both eyes in:

1. any direction
2. at any speed
3. at any frequency.

The same condition might appear to afflict readers of the heavier neurological texts, as they try in vain to grapple with the analyses and subdivisions of these tiny excursions into columns of minutiae that weary the memory and defeat reason.

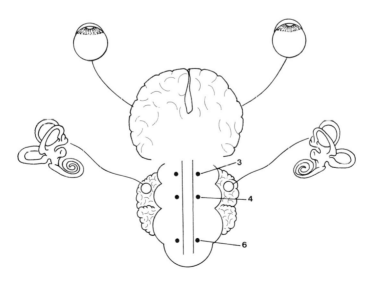

Fig. 19.1 A non-scale diagram of the elements which control voluntary and involuntary eye movements. Nystagmus is a parody of normality that ranges from defects in ocular fixation through paralysis of the extraocular movements to malfunction in the brain stem, cerebellum and vestibular apparatus.

Nystagmus occurs when some lesion induces a dysfunction in the normal mechanisms that initiate or modify ocular movements.

The third, fourth and sixth cranial nerves, linked to each other and to their fellows across the brain stem by the medial longitudinal bundles, control the six muscles which in turn control each eye.

Several factors control the nerves:

1. *Vision*: the eye fixes on objects of interest, provided the transparent tissues are transparent, there is no great defect in focus and the normal pathways from the retina to the conscious brain are intact.

   At a subconscious level other mechanisms can modify and even override instructions from above.
2. The *otoliths* give information about the position of the head in space.
3. The *semicircular canals* give information about movement of the head in space.
4. The *cerebellum* via the *vestibular nuclei* imposes a fine restraint on the natural coarseness of eye movements, as indeed it does in any other muscular activity – a mysterious mechanism, like so many other human faculties, appreciated only when it has ceased to function properly.

The cause of nystagmus may therefore lie either in the eye or in the brain. Since most of the controlling elements lie in the latter, then most of the lesions must lie there also. Unfortunately they are not always found.

All eyes with nystagmus move in a way that their possessor does not intend. That they move is invariably more important than how they move. There are, however, two circumstances where the nature of the movement makes the diagnosis.

Ocular nystagmus

A child born with some impairment of fixation, be it due to corneal opacity, congenital cataract or albinism, has no mechanism to hold the eye still in any position of gaze.

The eyes, therefore, develop a pendulum searching movement for a point of rest that forever eludes them.

The speed and amplitude of the movements are equal in all directions.

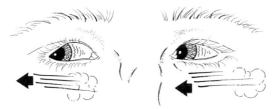

Fig. 19.2   End-point is the most common nystagmus. To one side then the other means exhaustion, debility, intoxication. To one side only could mean a partial sixth nerve palsy. The movements must be pushed to their limits or else the end point will not be reached.

End-point nystagmus

In states of general fatigue and languor, people may find it difficult to maintain their chosen ocular position in extremes of lateral gaze. The eyes keep drifting back to the centre and the person corrects this drift with a fast movement back to the original lateral position.

This fast movement is not without purpose.

It has to be noted that this end-point drift occurs only in lateral gaze and never in the straight ahead position. When the eyes move to either side, then the direction of the fast movement changes with them.

The unrestricted consumption of intoxicants can produce the same condition.

If end-point nystagmus occurs in one eye only then it cannot reasonably be considered the result of a systemic cause. There must be a local reason and it may well be the first sign of a frank sixth nerve palsy.

Long-standing nystagmus

There is usually someone on hand to confirm someone else's reputation for wandering eyes. In such cases, the patient's evident survival must show that, although the disease may be uncertain, life expectancy certainly is not.

Latent nystagmus

As the name implies, the condition is present only when a dominant eye is covered. Movement is of a roving searching quality and not greater in one direction than another.

Nystagmus of recent onset

Generally, the eye twitching is one of an abundance of signs that make the observation of nystagmus merely an interesting addition.

Occasionally, however, nystagmus may be the presenting feature.

Intracranial nystagmus

The movements here are not of equal speed. There is a fast component and a slow component, and the eyes may jerk in as many directions as the eyes can move.

Analysing these various components, neurologists can occasionally locate which part of the brain is at fault. The rest of us should be content with something less. Intracranial nystagmus divides into those of long standing and those of recent onset. The real question then is not how are the eyes twitching, but how recently did they begin to twitch?

Ataxic nystagmus

Some defect in the medial longitudinal bundle – usually demyelination – has an asymmetric effect on each eye. While one fails to adduct, the other fails to remain still – almost a grotesque caricature of brain-stem control over convergence and movements in parallel.

Cerebellar nystagmus

The cerebellum is the great coordinator. It does not initiate actions, it smooths them. When it fails, the eyes jerk coarsely, as do muscles elsewhere in the body.

Posterior fossa tumour

Cerebellar jerks may be the first sign of tumour in children who are symptomless in all other ways. It must be distinguished from:

1. ocular nystagmus – where the eyes do not jerk
2. latent nystagmus – where one eye jerks only when the other is covered.

Parental observation of recent onset should eliminate any tragic misdiagnosis, although the certain malignant pathology must temper any pleasure that might come to us from being right.

Spasmus nutans

Very occasionally a 6-month-old baby embarks on a strange course of apparently pointless head nodding, while jerking the eyes around in an asymmetric and equally pointless way.

Since so much else of one's behaviour at 6 months might appear to the adult to be pointless, there is nothing to be gained by trying to find a reason for it, especially if the child would appear to be happy and normal in every other way. The habit is of no consequence and the child will happily return to normality within a few months, before investigation has put this likelihood at risk.

SUMMARY

That the eyes move and how long they have moved is more important than how they move.

1. Searching equal movements of long standing – ocular nystagmus due to poor fixation.
2. Eyes which fail to hold the extremes of gaze, drifting into the middle before flicking back in their attempt at direction – end-point nystagmus:
   a. fatigue
   b. intoxication
   c. general ability
   d. sixth nerve palsy if unilateral.

Nystagmus of recent origin must be taken seriously and must be explained.

Intracranial causes are to be found in:

1. the brain stem – demyelination
2. the cerebellum – usually tumour, most often in childhood.

20. Eye disorders in childhood

The eye of a child is not all that different from that of an adult. However there are one or two features which justify a separate chapter. Extreme youth must give more prominence to congenital disorders. The growing sclera is capable of growing more than it ought to under the influence of intraocular pressure; the lens nucleus is still soft and the pathways of central vision have yet to be rendered functional.

The real problem with little patients is to get near enough for an adequate look at the eyes, the alleged malfunction of which is usually the subject of some second-hand history. The aim of the seven signs for children is the same as in adults. If it differs, it is only because children are not prepared to sit still for long enough to let us get to the end.

Vision

Snellen testing is not practical when people are too young to read or too mulish to want to.

At a crude level it is possible to get some sort of clue that a child can see, even if the response is a screaming fit when we pick up an instrument so full of menace as a torch. An element of subtlety can be introduced, and indeed some degree of macular function detected, by the ability to distinguish between pictures of teddy bears or houses or cowboys or policemen.

The most subtle technique, bypassing the need for letters or any desire to look at them, is called the Catford Drum. It carries dots on its side, the equivalent of the whole range of letters on the Snellen chart, and it oscillates. The eyes will follow the oscillation with an involuntary movement, which keeps returning to pick up the dot as it comes back again. This phenomenon is called opto-kinetic nystagmus.

Precise examination of the eyes may call for a general anaesthetic, but some elements of the seven signs can be snatched, and indeed some must be, before anaesthesia obliterates them.

Cornea and pupil

All we need to look at them is a good torch and enough time between spasms.

Raised intraocular pressure in the child – infantile glaucoma (buphthalmos)

The anterior chamber in the developing eye is full of embryonic tissue that normally disappears but sometimes does not. Should these remnants block the aqueous flow then of course the intraocular pressure must rise and, as the pressure rises, so must the sclera stretch.

The result is a hazy cornea in a large eye which waters, dislikes the light and cannot see properly ,and which if neglected will eventually fail to see at all.

The early eye surgeons faced with something so apparently incurable did the only thing they could, which was to describe it in classical terms. The name buphthalmos implies similarity to the bovine eye – a similarity limited only to its dimensions.

Management

The treatment is surgical. Abnormal tissue can be swept away with a needle from a narrow angle, and normal drainage and normal vision should follow.

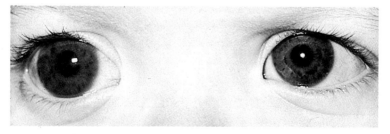

Fig. 20.1   Infantile glaucoma. A large cornea alone does not give the diagnosis. It should be cloudy as well, the IOP raised and a general anaesthetic may be necessary to prove the second (prompted by the first).

However, should the angle also be abnormal as part of an inherited defect, in which case an external drainage operation can make some attempt to establish aqueous flow. Such operations do not always succeed because the only healthy thing in these eyes is their fibrotic response to anything so outrageous as a deliberate fistula. Visual decline is then relentless.

Megalocornea

Not all large globes are pathological. It should be remembered that the 2-year-old cornea is already adult-sized, giving it that magnificent lustre that excites a bitter-sweet regret in withered adults who contemplate their own childhood portraits.

Some of these eyes are even bigger still- megalocornea – but in all circumstances a normal cornea and a normal pupil distinguish them from the eye of infantile 'glaucoma'.

Retinoblastoma

This growth is fortunately as rare as it is malignant – occurring once in rather more than 20 000 live births.

From its favourite site of origin in the posterior retina, it rapidly fills the vitreous with tumour seedlings – which whiten the normally black pupil. It is this feature, and perhaps the occasional squint, rather than visual loss, which catches parental notice.

Most cases present before the age of 3 and there is a one-in-three chance that both eyes may be affected.

Management

Enucleation is obligatory for large tumours, but smaller ones may be attacked by a combination of radiotherapy and chemotherapy – both methods curing a large percentage of those unfortunate youngsters.

In known families, the heredity appears to be an autosomal dominant with 80% penetrance. In practical terms this means that half the children will carry the trait, and of this half four out of five will suffer the disease.

Where there is no family history, it seems however that most cases are sporadic. More and more of these children survive to become parents themselves and their offspring do not seem to demonstrate any dominant hereditary pattern.

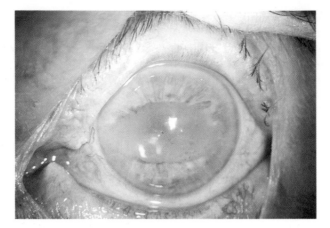

Fig. 20.2   Band keratopathy. The cornea may develop surface opacities in response to long-term intraocular inflammation.

Iritis and Still's disease

Iritis complicates both adult and juvenile rheumatism, although the complications are more damaging in children simply because they have more time to be so.

The condition smoulders, poisoning the aqueous as the years go by. Corticosteroids, both topical and systemic, only delay the decline into cataract, a rise in pressure secondary to iritis, failed operations for the same, band-shaped scars across the front of the cornea and finally visual collapse.

Fortunately it is as rare as it is hard to treat.

Coloboma

The eyeball and lower lid have a single seam of union running from the optic disc forwards along the lower nasal meridian. Failure of this seam to close perfectly is called a coloboma.

It may range from a negligible notch in the eyelid to a total absence of everything but sclera along the line of failure closure.

No treatment is indicated except when a retinal detachment complicates the issue.

Retinopathy of prematurity

The identical clinical picture, under the name of retrolental fibroplasia, has been identified as due to excessive exposure to oxygen after birth. It was quietly sliding into the chapters of history when the neonatologist resurrected it under its present title.

With their skill in rescuing babies of decreasing birth-weight and increasing prematurity, it created a dilemma that makes great demands on the parents' emotions and on the ophthalmological services.

In normal circumstances blood vessels go in an ordered pattern in the retina from the retina to the ora serrata. When this order is disturbed the threat of blindness can be added to all the other possible organ defects facing these tiny children.

Grade 1

At its least severe a line of demarcation forms between the peripheral vascular retina and the advancing blood vessels.

Grade 2

This line may acquire a third dimension, heaping up into a ridge.

Grade 3

With the usual ocular behaviour of limited response, the anoxic retina responds with the development of abnormal fragile new blood vessels. Grade 3 is the watershed of this disease. Spontaneous regression may remove the risk of blindness but continued progression without treatment, and indeed even with treatment, can proceed to bilateral tractional retinal detachment.

Management

Management consists of regular retinal examination through the dilated pupil of all premature babies of very low birth-weight. To begin with these examinations can be carried out only in the exhausting temperature of the neonatal intensive care unit during the first 12 weeks of life.

New vessels progressing to more new vessels are taken as the indication to intervene. This intervention is based on the same principles as that for diabetic retinopathy (the limited response again). The peripheral avascular retina is subjected to inflammation using either cold (cryotherapy) or heat (laser photocoagulation) both under general anaesthesia in the neonatal unit.

It is now accepted that prompt adequate treatment can greatly reduce the incidence of blindness due to this unhappy condition. Its existence, however, encapsulates neatly the medical dilemma that the elimination of one major scourge can give birth to more than one in its wake.

As for the rest, most childhood disease can be accounted for by squint and infections of the external eye. Thereafter we have to consider a catalogue of rarities involving malformation of the skull, of the eye and its adjacent structures, and even rarer conditions such as gargoylism.

SUMMARY

Children generally see no reason why they should cooperate in anything so unpleasant as an ophthalmic examination, even if the seven signs do not require much time. We may be forced occasionally to consider general anaesthesia. There is a natural reluctance to consider anaesthesia but it would be tragic to miss anything treatable because of that reluctance.

21. Squint

Much of our capacity to change direction of gaze is provided by the head swivelling and nodding upon the neck. After that it is up to the eyes to extend that range of vision.

Both eyes normally move with each other in parallel when they are focused in the distance. However, they have to move against each other out of parallel when they converge to focus on something near – a reflex but recently acquired in the process of evolution and often the first to vanish when the shocks of existence become too much to bear.

Six muscles supplied by three nerves are responsible for the movements of each eye. Since the third nerve innervates much more than the fourth and sixth, it makes more sense to consider the nerves in reverse order.

1. The *sixth nerve* (*abducent*) sends impulses to the lateral rectus which moves the eye outwards.
2. The *fourth nerve* (*trochlear*) sends impulses to the superior oblique which turns the eye downwards most effectively when it is in the converged position for reading.
3. The *third nerve* (*oculomotor*) sends impulses to all the other muscles. In addition it innovates the levator which raises the upper lid and is the outflow limb of the pupil reflex carrying impulses for constriction in response to:
    a. light
    b. accommodation.

The entire arrangement is designed to point both eyes at the same time at the same object to achieve perception and depth. This faculty is what we call binocular vision.

Its influence can be neatly demonstrated when someone tries to catch a bouncing rugby ball with both eyes open and then with one eye closed or risks the paintwork of a new car with an identical visual experiment.

Eyes which squint belong to quite separate groups:

1. those without binocular vision
2. those with binocular vision.

The distinction is critical.

In the first group the eyes cannot be used at the same time because they are pointing in different directions. The result is the alternating use of either eye or the habitual use of one eye, whilst the central vision of the other lapses into amblyopia (lazy eye).

The second group do see with both eyes at the same time, because the brain has learned to interpret their simultaneous flow of essentially similar images. Separation of these eyes, classically by a paralysed muscle, will produce a simultaneous flow of wholly dissimilar images.

Each eye will continue to see at the same time, but it will not see the same thing. The result is a bitter complaint of double vision.

EYES WITHOUT BINOCULAR VISION

Most squinting eyes squint because there is no binocular desire to lock them together – apparently parallel for distance and converged for reading. Other factors occasionally interfere.

Long-sighted eyes have to focus in the distance as they would for near. Because they are focusing as they would for near, they also converge as they would for near. Unfortunately if they do so while they are looking into the distance (when they should be straight) then the result is a convergent squint.

While central vision is still taking root, it can be just as easily uprooted. Rather than tolerate the confusion of double images the brain will suppress the instinctive desire for both eyes to work together. If the eyes end up equal, the suppression will alternate from one to the other. If the eyes become unequal, the child will favour the one which is easier to use – the one with the lesser spectacle error.

The longer suppression continues, the more difficult it will be to reverse and by the age of 5 reversal is usually impossible.

For this reason, squint must be discovered early. A child will not grow out of a squint. The price of neglect is the macular function of one eye.

At the other end of the scale there is a lower age limit below which examination will only confirm to little patients what they already instinctively knew, that hospitals are not to be tolerated. By the age of a year or 18 months, they might be persuaded to co-operate for a while and not to concentrate their entire minds on potato crisps, sticky drinks or simple evasion.

Because the whole point of treatment is to improve and maintain macular function, the second point in examination is to see if macular function is present. Most parents are prepared for cosmetic defects but the menace to the child's central vision can test their resilience, as indeed our explanations may test their comprehension. They may not recover sufficiently from either to cooperate in treatment.

The cover test

Eyes that squint deviate from each other at a fixed angle. When one is looking straight ahead, the other does not and the angle between them is the angle of the squint.

If the second eye can now be persuaded to look straight ahead, the first one will do so no longer and the angle between them remains the unchanged angle of the squint.

Habitual fixation with one eye does not alter this fact. It merely tells us that the macula on that side is too good ever to let go and give the other macula a chance. But the angle of the squint still remains a fixed angle between both eyes. The cover test is a manoeuvre to demonstrate this angle.

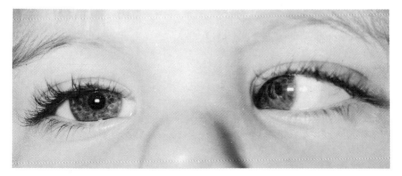

Fig. 21.1 The angle of squint is fixed no matter where the eyes move.

Because it is a test of fixation, we have to be sure that the child is in fact fixing. A torch is just another light and cannot be of any conceivable interest but a stick decorated with pictures like policemen, teddy bears and colourful birds might be more persuasive. These colourful images should have enough detail to stimulate near focus when an actual squint might then become quite obvious.

If we place a hand before first one eye and then the other we can demonstrate this horse-rein action of both eyes as they swing at their fixed angle.

The covered eye will move towards a squinting position whilst the uncovered eye will move to fix on the stick. This movement will be reversed when the hand covers the other eye and releases the first to take up fixation.

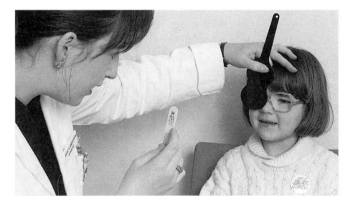

Fig. 21.2 The cover test.

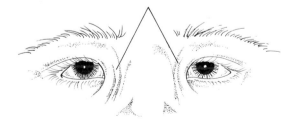

Fig. 21.3 Epicanthus gives the impression of a converging squint.

Genuine squint

— The eye movements tested separately will be full and equal
  with each other
— The eyes are set at the wrong angle
— The angle does not vary
— There is no muscle paralysis
— The child cannot complain of double vision.

Pseudosquint

Not all eyes that appear to squint are in fact squinting. An
apparent squint may be produced by facial asymmetry. Every face
has unequal sides; some are just more obvious than others.

Exaggerated skin folds from the upper lid to the nose (epicanthus), a racial characteristic of south-east Asian peoples but not of
others, can give the impression of convergence.

That these folds recede spontaneously has not prevented
impatient surgeons from attempting to hasten their recession.
And children, formerly tormented at school with the nickname of
'Slit-eyes' have been known to report tearfully the even more
fearful sobriquet of 'Scar-face'.

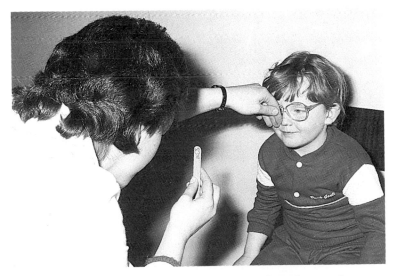

Fig. 21.4   Eyes without binocular vision. As one eye fixes, the second converges.
As the second eye fixes, the first converges. The angle remains the same.

Tests for binocular function

In orthoptic departments the exact angle of the squint and the grading of binocular function can be assessed using a synoptophore. Although this is subtle and accurate it is also the province of the orthoptic expert, which almost certainly excludes most eye surgeons.

There are simpler methods. The presence of three-dimensional vision can be proved when flat, polarized images spring to life when viewed through polarizing spectacles. The 'stereoscopic fly' is based on this principle and its cartoon characters should compete quite successfully for the attention of the average 2-year-old.

The cover test, although glibly discussed, is not always easy to do. If a child considered to squint turns out to have demonstrable binocular vision, then the chances are that there is no squint. Should one be present then the chances are that central vision will have developed equally already, which takes much of the urgency out of further treatment.

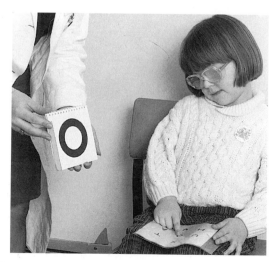

Fig. 21.5   Testing visual acuity.

Management

Nothing sensible can be done about a squint until any retinal abnormality is discovered and any spectacle error corrected. Neither is possible without dilatation of the pupil, which permits:

1. accurate refraction
2. fundal examination, where a constricting pupil is not added to the nightmare of a dodging head.

If a scar, for whatever reason, exists at the macula then subsequent orthoptic treatment will be fruitless and needless. It should also be remembered that sinister conditions like retinoblastoma or a retinal detachment may present as an eye squinting because fixation is lost.

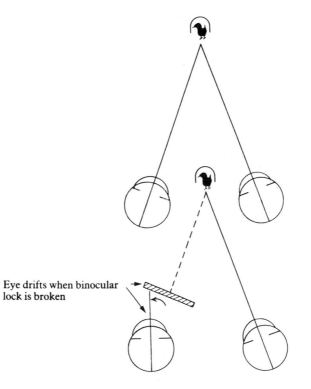

Eye drifts when binocular lock is broken

Fig. 21.6   Eyes with binocular vision. The cover–uncover test exposes eyes which want to point visually together, but physically find it difficult.

Once a frank deviation has been demonstrated, then the child has to be handed over to orthoptists who are well practised in wheedling information out of truculent toddlers. If the central vision of one eye be reduced even with appropriate glasses then they will set out on a course of patching. This involves occlusion of the good eye for some of the waking hours to force the poorer eye to drive a functional path through to the visual cortex.

Although these explanations may be conducted amidst smiling good-will it is mother who has to deal with all the tantrums and defiance during the period of occlusion. It is vital that this occlusion be carried out ruthlessly by a combination of cajolery and implacable disbelief in promises of good behaviour tomorrow if only the patch can come off today.

Treatment aims to establish equal macular vision. Once each eye is fixing alternately, then functional visual path to the brain is open. Should the central vision of one eye decline afterwards because the other eye is preferred, then this central vision can always be restored should it ever be needed because of this open pathway.

If the pathway has never been opened and macular vision therefore never established, then all the expensive intercessions so readily available to anxious and gullible parents will not make it do so.

Surgery

In some countries where medical treatment is not readily available or if available not welcomed, an imposing squint may be considered a token of military genius or at least as a delivery system for evil rays. Such prized qualities, often leading to tribal leadership, will not be lightly exchanged for a comely appearance.

When such prizes are not at stake, a deviation of any degree is generally regarded as a cosmetic defect, amenable to surgery before first-year school mates discover their talent for wounding nicknames.

Because there is no binocular lock, the eyes once straightened may continue to drift in time in the same direction and point outwards because the orbits point outwards anyway. Such consecutive diversion, as it is called, can be reversed by further surgery some years later.

Amblyopia

The lazy eye must rival glaucoma and lasers in retinal detachment for top place in the popular misconception ratings.

A lazy eye is a normal eye with perfect field vision but less than perfect central vision. Such imperfection dates from early life when macular development has been hampered.

A squint can of course hamper development of the macula but does not always do so; so can ptosis, congenital cataract and spectacle errors that have not been corrected.

The eye may squint. A squinting eye may be lazy but a straight eye may be lazy also.

Anisometropic amblyopia

This mouthful is the technical name given when central visual development is arrested (amblyopia, lazy eye) in one eye because the eyes are too different to work together.

A cataract removed from one eye in later life and uncorrected prevents both eyes from uniting in binocular vision but clearly cannot undevelop a developed macula. However, an undeveloped macula is in danger if the eyes are so discrepant from birth. Early correction allows them to adapt. If such correction has been rejected or neglected then we have a little longer to play with, perhaps even into the early teens, to force a lazy eye into action by patching its normal fellow.

EYES WITH BINOCULAR VISION

After full binocular vision has formed, anything that makes one visual axis deviate from its fellow will result in two distinct images which separate in direct proportion to the deviation. There are three conditions which result in this and in all of them the symptoms will vanish when one eye is covered:

1. extraocular muscle paralysis
2. latent squint
3. convergence weakness.

Extraocular muscles

Whatever the underlying cause, a paralysed muscle in a conscious patient with developed binocular vision must produce double vision. Patients frequently complain of double vision when they really mean blurred vision. A thoughtful history should make the distinction clear. It should also begin to sift through the list of possible causes.

Double vision in a young person must always be taken seriously, whether it is of sudden onset or of languid onset. Even in the absence of headache, serious conditions such as an intracranial aneurysm must be assumed until disproved.

In the older patient a sudden onset usually means a vascular accident in the brain stem.

Long-standing conditions should bridle our diagnostic flights of fancy with the irrefutable observation that the patient has clearly survived to tell the tale.

Examination

That the seven signs should be applied goes without saying.

The eye movements should be tested also not as part of a separate ophthalmic examination but as part of the general cranial nerve examination, which can and should be completed.

Should the double vision be due to a paralysed muscle, separation of the double images will increase when that paralysed muscle is called upon to undertake its natural movement.

Investigation must sensibly include:

1. urinalysis for sugar
2. an estimate of blood pressure
3. a full blood count
4. radiography, including CT scanning of the skull.

If serious intracranial disease is suspected then the proper course of action is always referral to a neurosurgeon.

Pathological basis

Any disease from the brain stem to the orbit may cause a muscle to function poorly. The commonest must be trauma but viral inflammation of the cranial nerves is more common than might be expected.

Of the intracranial lesions, aneurysm or tumour must be considered before any other in younger age groups whilst diabetes, hypertension and arteriosclerosis have to be first on the list in the older age groups.

Fluctuating double vision worsening towards the end of the day is almost diagnostic of myasthenia gravis, whilst a muscle palsy as part of an unconnected catalogue of signs must raise the spectre of demyelination.

Thiamine deficiency can have an equally widespread influence, dislocating the mind and the nervous control of the muscles from the eyes to the legs.

Latent squint

In nobody are the eyes absolutely straight. There is always a slight hidden deviation, normally overcome by an irresistible binocular lock. Such deviations become significant only when the eyes would prefer to separate from each other more than the binocular lock can tolerate.

Symptoms of fleeting double vision and difficulty in depth perception depend on how quickly such people can pull their eyes together.

If another stress is added then the lock may just break apart altogether. A classic example of this came to light during the war when certain pilots found it impossible to judge their height from the runway – an understandable lapse of judgment if enemy aircraft were prowling about.

The cover-uncover test

We can demonstrate that everyone has a latent squint using this test. It tells us two things:

1. how far the eye has to travel to get back into position
2. how well and how quickly it travels.

Just occasionally the lateral rectus trembling on the brink of frank palsy can give the impression of a latent convergent squint. That it is of recent and possibly sudden onset should alert us to such a possibility.

Management

As uncorrected errors of refraction can sometimes exaggerate a deviation, the first step must be to correct them.

In the absence of so simple a cure, exercises for the extraocular muscles can sometimes produce subjective improvement whilst leaving the deviation very much as it was.

When deviations prove too much for these simple remedies, then the position of the eyes themselves may be altered. Not infrequently, such a threat makes previously scorned exercises appear just the treatment that the patient had in mind.

Convergence weakness

The convergence reflex, our most recent acquisition during evolution, is frequently the first to disintegrate under stress. What might be considered as stress will vary according to one's interests, but the thought of studying on a hot summer evening or the embarrassment at imminent exposure at an examination may induce students from time to time to develop double vision for near objects.

They lose their capacity to converge the eyes, find grave difficulty in reading and thus produce an irresistible excuse for idling.

There is no extraocular muscle palsy. The eyes can look both right and left but cannot converge to read. The complaint can be verified by the development of double images with a fixation stick before it has come within the normal reading distance.

Management

If general health is good and muscle movements normal, then simple exercises at home can help bring the convergence point nearer to the nose.

In those golden days before package holidays took over, old textbooks on refraction would recommend a winter on skis by the Jungfrau as an essential part of the cure. The authors may have cynically reckoned that the inevitable broken leg would bring about a swift recovery in convergence as the only available relief from boredom.

SUMMARY

1. The eyes drift apart when either is covered.
2. In most people, this latent drift is kept in check by the powerful binocular lock.
3. In some people a pronounced drift may with added stress become more pronounced and break the binocular lock.
4. In all people with developed binocular vision, a paralysed extraocular muscle must break the binocular lock – especially when that lock is called upon to act.
5. In most children who squint there is no binocular lock.

22. Trauma

Injuries, no matter where they strike in the body, have two aspects. The first and obvious one is the instant damage. The second is the possible long-term complication, either at the site of injury or at a more distant site.

Apart from a few well-defined conditions demanding urgent specialist attention, anyone familiar with the craft of suturing can attend to most ocular injuries. They are skin lacerations, and ocular only because they happen to be in the upper face.

Injuries become the province of the ophthalmic specialist in four main categories:

1. intraocular foreign body
2. injury to the eyeball
3. injury to the eyelid
4. injury to the orbit.

The only equipment necessary to evaluate the damage is a good torch. The other eye may serve as a normal control.

INTRAOCULAR FOREIGN BODY

In any violence involving the eye, a foreign body within the globe should always be suspected. Fragments of steel from hammer or chisel or pieces of shattered windscreen are common culprits. It is always wise to ask if anything was travelling fast enough to penetrate the eye.

However the failure to judge the value of goggles, or the value of seat belts, may extend to an equal failure to judge the speed of any possible penetrants.

Close examination of the eyeball may show an entry point, iris distortion being a helpful guide. But a fragment entering the limbus could leave the eye looking entirely normal until its ill effects become obvious some time later.

If an eye hospital is close at hand then referral is the correct approach. However, in remoter districts a radiograph of the orbits is a useful preliminary. Absence of orbital opacities could save a needless journey, whereas a positive demonstration of these could save the eye.

Intraocular metal fragments left long enough in situ will oxidize and deposit metal salts throughout the globe. Ferrous metals used to be extracted with magnets, but to lift them out precisely with forceps is preferable to dragging them out over the delicate structures with a magnet. Non-magnetic metals would demand forceps extraction by choice anyway, and the eye may be luckier for that.

The lens, indifferent to the exact nature of the penetrating agent, may develop a cataract if its capsule has been violated.

INJURY TO THE EYEBALL

Damage may be laceration, contusion or chemical.

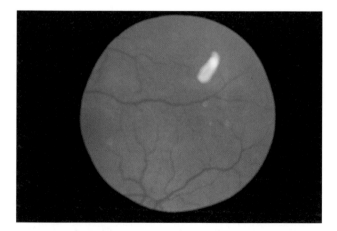

Fig. 22.1   Intraocular brass foreign body – the unhappy result of a shooting expedition. In time, metal, reacting with the ocular fluids, would deposit salts throughout the ocular tissues, with subsequent total destruction of the globe. Although these injuries are often sterile, early extraction reduces the very real danger of intraocular infection and is technically easier through a transparent lens.

Laceration

This is easily recognized and it is equally easy for infection to get in and, with careless handling, easy for the contents of the eye to get out.

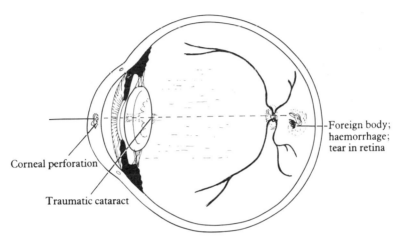

Corneal perforation

Traumatic cataract

Foreign body;
haemorrhage;
tear in retina

Fig. 22.2   An intraocular foreign body is not always obvious. A history may have to be extracted from the patient with as much difficulty as the foreign body.

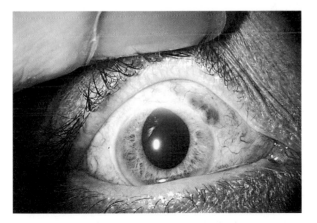

Fig. 22.3   Iris prolapse. There might be a slight hint of pupil-peaking towards the 2 o'clock meridian. Trauma is the most likely cause, either in a healthy eye or in one weakened by recent surgery.

Systemic antibiotics might be the first line of action against the first, whilst avoiding pressure on the globe is a sensible precaution against the second – even after the laceration has been sutured.

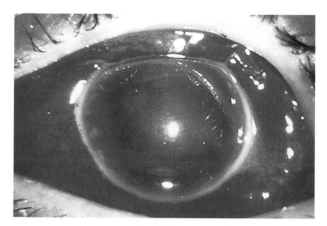

Fig. 22.4   Traumatic subconjunctival haemorrhage. Although the conjunctival redness appears fearful, the absence of vascular markings indicates the existence of haemorrhage. Haemorrhage within the anterior chamber is a surer indicator of serious ocular damage, which may involve the drainage meshwork, the lens or the peripheral retina.

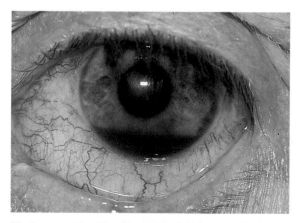

Fig. 22.5   Hyphaema – blood in the anterior chamber, usually the result of trauma. The eye is irritable and the secondary bleed can 1) fill the anterior chamber, 2) block the drain, 3) raise the pressure and 4) stain the cornea.

Contusion

The imagination can supply a catalogue of possible agents, but ball games and fisticuffs must rank high on the list. Trauma anywhere causes bleeding, instant damage to vital structures and long-term inflammatory fibrotic damage to everything.

Blood in the anterior chamber

Commonly called hyphaema, this is recognized by fluid level which settles out rather like blood in an ESR tube. Blood products silting into the trabecular meshwork can raise the intraocular pressure.

If the hyphaema is total, the inevitable raised pressure squeezes blood into the corneal stroma, where it leaves a permanent stain.

Management

Bed rest can prevent the secondary haemorrhage that seems to lead to this catastrophe. Topical corticosteroids will suppress inflammation.

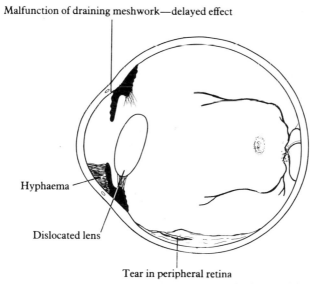

Malfunction of draining meshwork—delayed effect

Hyphaema

Dislocated lens

Tear in peripheral retina

Fig. 22.6 A blow severe enough to cause hyphaema can also dislocate the lens, tear the retina and raise the intraocular pressure – but not always immediately.

If the hyphaema is to be evacuated surgically the inevitable pressure rise must be controlled in the usual way.

Long term

Later developments from blunt trauma may show in later years. Glaucoma can follow, secondary to the fibrosis of the drainage angle; retinal tears sustained from the original blow can bring about a detachment at any time, so long after in fact that the connection may not be suspected. A lens that survives dislocation may not survive cataract formation.

A good rule is that a blow sufficient to cause hyphaemia can rupture the globe, dislocate the lens, tear the peripheral retina and raise the intraocular pressure. The first step to diagnosis and management is to consider these things possible.

Chemical

The range could be bewildering, but strong acids or alkalis are familiar on the industrial scene and have long been used as a silent substitute for the gun in the prosecution of villainous stratagems.

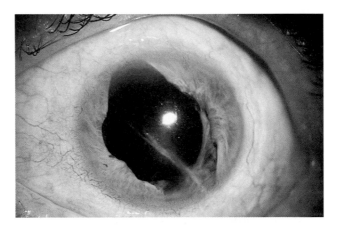

Fig. 22.7   Trauma to the anterior segment. This eye demonstrates a corneal scar which at one time was probably the entry point of a foreign body which penetrated the lens. The lens is now gone, leaving fragments of capsule. The irregular pupil tells us that iris has to be sacrificed to preserve the integrity of the remaining anterior segment.

Both chemicals cause lethal damage. They distort the eyelids (causing them to adhere to the eye), turn in the lashes, cause opacity of the cornea and scarify the drainage angle.

Alkali injuries are the more sinister, in that they sink deeper into the eye, causing more complicated disturbance than do acids, whose coagulating action limits penetration.

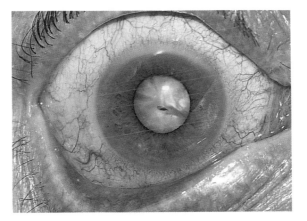

Fig. 22.8   Traumatic cataract. Whatever the insult, the lens has but one response, namely to develop a cataract. The ciliary injection, dominant around the corneoscleral limbus, indicates a deep-seated inflammation – probably iritis.

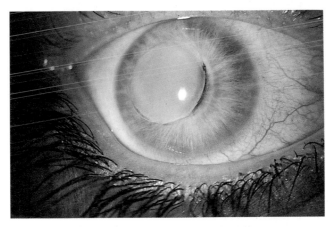

Fig. 22.9   Lens dislocated into anterior chamber – already affecting vision and threatening pressure control and the deep corneal surface.

The short-term management is to flood the eye with water as soon as possible.

The long-term management is the attempted reversal of all the ghastly complications, and indeed the attempts do not always succeed.

INJURY TO THE EYELID

There are two particular types which demand specialist attention within 24 hours. These are lacerations involving:

1. the lid margin
2. the lower canaliculus.

In the short term we must check that the lacerating agent has not damaged more than the eyelid. If the globe is intact, it will in the short term suffer irritation from exposure which in the longer term will lead to infection and the inevitable replacement of specialised tissue with functionless connective tissue.

As the eye is happiest when shut, closure of the lids with adhesive tape over lubricating ointment will relieve the discomfort and prevent further damage within.

In the long term the integrity of the external alliance demands accurate surgical restoration of the eyelid margin – presenting a continuous rounded edge to the corneal surface with the lashes pointing the other way.

Long-term management demands accurate surgical apposition. A notch at the injury site can result in permanent intractable watering, not to mention what exposure or maverick lashes can do to the corneal epithelium.

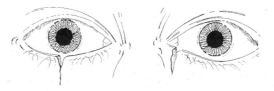

Fig. 22.10 Laceration of the lid margins must take precedence over everything except actual laceration of the globe itself.

The watering that follows canalicular injuries is distressing but not as distressing as the increased watering which results from damage to the upper canaliculus during failed surgery on the lower.

INJURY TO THE ORBIT

A blow-out fracture of the orbital floor is a popular weekend injury, often when the victim's perception is not at its best. A savage blow forces the orbital contents into the maxillary sinus, where the eye muscles will be trapped by bony fragments. The tethered eye will move neither upwards or downwards, and if the condition is neglected it never will again.

Tethered eye movements and loss of sensation over the distribution of the infraorbital nerve between the orbital margin and the lip are classic signs. Settling oedema may demonstrate that the eye has sunk in comparison with its fellow.

If the swollen lids can be forced open, it is possible to run through the ophthalmic ritual, checking the three visions, the cornea, the pupil and the anterior chamber, which may be compared with the normal fellow eye.

Radiographic examination will confirm or refute any clinical impression.

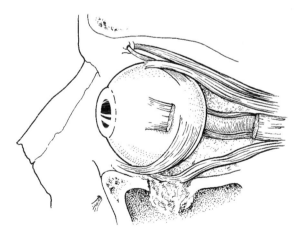

Fig. 22.11   If the orbit and the eye are too swollen to reveal detail, loss of sensation over the cheek would suggest trapping of the maxillary nerve in the orbital floor. A blow sufficient to rupture the orbital floor can also do fearful things to the globe itself.

It is necessary to elevate the contents of the orbit and keep them in position with a plate of silicone rubber to make good the defect in the orbital floor.

Sympathetic ophthalmitis

A penetrating injury, particularly one involving the lens iris and ciliary body, can stimulate the production of circulating antibodies to normal eye tissue. These antibodies fail to recognize the eyes as 'self' and, brought into being by one, may end by attacking both.

The result is a smouldering pan-uveitis, with all the signs of iritis in the anterior chamber – swollen retinal veins and inflammatory cells in the vitreous – to indicate that the posterior part of the uvea has been involved as well.

Because the condition is happily rare, it is not easy to establish guidelines in practice. But renewed pain in a red, watering eye would be accepted as a symptom that should not be ignored.

Should the exciting eye be damaged beyond the hope of useful vision, then enucleation may save the fellow from any involvement.

The dilemma starts when the inflamed eye has useful vision as well as all the signs of sympathetic ophthalmitis. We cannot remove it because it may end up the better eye.

Because the condition is so rare, percentage incidence means little, but it tends not to happen in the first few weeks following injury, because presumably the antibodies have been prepared. If it has not followed after 3 months, then its chances of following at all diminish with every day that passes.

SUMMARY

Damage to the eyelids risks the integrity of their margin or the patency of the lower canaliculi. Injury to the globe, apart from its obvious features, may in the long term result in cataract, chronic secondary glaucoma and retinal detachment.

An intraocular foreign body is always possible, no matter how convincing may be the history to the contrary.

A blow-out fracture of the orbit may not be apparent until settling oedema reveals what has happened.

Any penetrating eye injury, including surgery, can give rise to sympathetic ophthalmitis.

23. Proptosis

When the available space in the orbit ceases to be adequate to contain the eyeball as well as the orbital contents, then the eye will advance, pushing the lids aside until its prominence persuades us to make a diagnosis of proptosis.

Another name – exophthalmos -means very much the same thing, but has tended to be reserved for proptosis due to thyroid disease, when the orbital contents change not only their size but also their character.

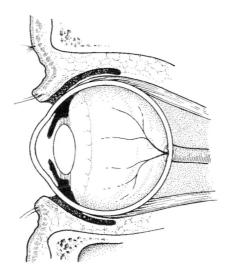

Fig. 23.1 Alien material in the orbit can compress and destroy the optic nerve and also push the eye beyond the capacity of the lids to cover it.

There are two basic problems. The first is that the condition is potentially life-threatening if the cause of the proptosis turns out to be malignant. The second is that it is eye-threatening for two reasons:

1. exposure of the cornea
2. compression of the optic nerve at the apex of the orbit.

AETIOLOGY

A wide-ranging collection of disease processes, from lymphomas to simple trauma, can fill the orbital space with unhealthy or alien tissue. In practice, fortunately, the permutations are reduced to a small workable collection – the most common being thyroid disease which, contrary to popular belief, may be unilateral in some 20% of cases.

SYMPTOMS

A mass within the orbit, no matter what its cause, can produce symptoms that fit into the general ophthalmic pattern:

—   it may cause pain
—   it certainly causes a change in appearance
—   pressure on the eye or optic nerve may distort or diminish vision
—   the globe may be pushed beyond the capacity of the muscles to maintain binocular vision, resulting in double vision
—   exposure of the cornea can result in watering.

Once again, here is an example of widely different disease processes converging on the same clinical condition, using up all the available symptoms without particularly leading us to a certain diagnosis.

EXAMINATION

Deflection of the eye to one side would suggest a local mass – for example, a lacrimal gland tumour. Simple advance of the globe – axial proptosis – whilst it may follow a diffuse infiltration of the globe, may also result from an optic nerve glioma.

Thyroid

An overactive gland is popularly associated with prominent eye. That restoration of the euthyroid state may in fact be associated with even more prominent eyes is not so well known.

Thyroid disease takes us into the field of baffling endocrine malfunction. However, an exophthalmos-inducing immunoglobulin has now been quite clearly identified.

Retraction of the upper eyelid, exaggerating the eyeball protrusion, is a classic distinguishing feature of thyroid-induced proptosis.

In the general flutter of sympathetic overactivity, the autonomic levator acts independently of its fellow.

Mucopolysaccharides deposited within the orbit and within the extramacular muscles push the eye forward and limit the ability of the muscles to maintain normal movements. Occasionally, an oedematous conjunctiva may herniate and strangulate through tight eyelids.

A confident clinical diagnosis of thyroid disease is not always supported by abnormal blood levels of the various thyroid factors. Even in their absence it is probably still the likely cause.

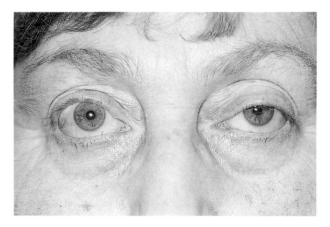

Fig. 23.2 Exophthalmos. Accumulation of abnormal tissue within the orbit takes up space normally occupied by the eye, which protrudes. The dangers are compression of the optic nerve at the orbital apex and exposure of the cornea.

Investigations, though, should include orbital radiographs, which sometimes demonstrate bony erosion or widening of the optic foramina. A full blood count cannot be regarded as a complicated investigation.

However, a collection of negative findings at this point leaves us impaled on the horns of a diagnostic dilemma. Should we observe a proptosed eye without diagnosis or threaten the same eye by searching for one – the biopsy of which may leave a nerve palsy in its track and produce a nightmare smudge of tissues for the histologist to equivocate over?

There is much to be said for doing nothing, measuring regularly the lack of change in both types of vision, corneal exposure and the appearance of the optic nerve head.

When increasing symptoms and signs make a diagnosis an urgent necessity, then the CT scan may provide enormous information about the diagnosis and the orbital contents without damaging them.

Pseudotumour

An imposing title for indecision. It looks like a unilateral tumour but in fact it is grumbling granulomatous inflammation. If biopsy be ventured, there might be one or two ambiguous differences from other more unpleasant disorders.

Resolution with high doses of systemic corticosteroids can sometimes produce the same diagnosis by inference, as well as clinical improvement without recourse to the knife.

Acute proptosis

Carotico-cavernous sinus fistula

Amongst a catalogue of rarities, this must be the most important. It may follow fracture at the base of the skull or, more rarely, spontaneous rupture of the carotid artery within the cavernous sinus.

Its clinical features arise entirely from high pressure arterial blood pulsing in a low-tension system – the most obvious of which is the superior ophthalmic vein.

The conjunctival vessels can be seen to be widely dilated, whilst dilatation of the rest is apparent from the swollen lids and protruding eye.

The cause is clear because the proptosis is pulsatile.

Orbital cellulitis

The acute infection of the orbit, either as a blood-borne disorder or as a result of an adjacent sinusitis, results in all the local signs of inflammation as well as a systemic fever.

Cavernous sinus thrombosis

This rare and devastating bilateral catastrophe produces gross venous congestion and disturbance of the third, fourth, fifth and sixth cranial nerves, which traverse the wall of the sinus on their way to the orbit.

The patient will be clearly prostrated by a severe illness and this is no time to debate trifles at length by the bedside.

As both conditions are happily rare, it is not always easy to stand firm upon textbook descriptions, which happen more often in textbooks than they do in reality. However, a unilateral condition with normal pupils in a reasonably well, though fevered, patient should make the distinction of orbital cellulitis from the more severely disabling cavernous sinus thrombosis.

MANAGEMENT

The aim must be to preserve both eye and life, though in childhood malignancy neither of these is always possible. The cause should be removed, but if it cannot then its ill effects should be curbed. Long-term function, of course, means the passage of light through a transparent cornea to a retina served by a healthy optic nerve.

At a simple level, corneal exposure may be treated with artificial tears or by small plastic procedures to narrow the palpebral fissure. Diplopia due to muscle palsies does not always respond to surgical alteration of their position because the muscles themselves are diseased. A black patch over either eye may remove the symptoms and at the end of the day may be more effective than surgery.

At a higher level the threat of gross corneal exposure or optic nerve compression may require an ENT surgeon to allow the orbital contents to expand medially and downwards or a neurosurgeon to liberate them above.

Thereafter we must always balance the danger of the condition against the danger of the investigation. Many such eyes remain unchanged for years, defying all attempts at a diagnosis while the patient's survival demonstrates how wise it was in the first place to leave well alone.

Looking at old family photographs may be a simple way of proving that a recent complaint of proptosis is merely a recent observation of something that has been going on for a long time.

SUMMARY

Any material taking up space normally occupied by the eye will push it forward through the lids.

The most likely cause in adults is thyroid dysfunction, even after endocrine balance has been restored.

In children, malignant disease comes first on a short list.

At any age, rapid onset is rare. Of these:

1. an *arteriovenous fistula* is pulsatile
2. *orbital cellulitis* is unilateral, accompanied by fever
3. *cavernous sinus thrombosis* is devastating and bilateral.

The danger to the eye from the simple causes is corneal exposure and optic nerve compression.

24. Examinations: how to pass them

The popular cameo of an examination is a confrontation, a duel between some monstrous creation of Roald Dahl and some helpless student whose life of innocent pleasure has left but little time for study. And behind the scenes, nights of frenzy and huge textbooks which defend their contents against a determined attempt to convert them into a last minute imitation of scholarship.

The resultant failure, or scraped pass, then confirms the belief that examinations are just short of armed combat and that they can be passed only by hoodwinking the examiner with a parade of small-print obscurities. In fact, examiners are not so easily taken in and most candidates who fail do so because they have not grasped the large-print principles.

Any examination can be turned into an easy canter by a little understanding of how it is structured, an understanding of how

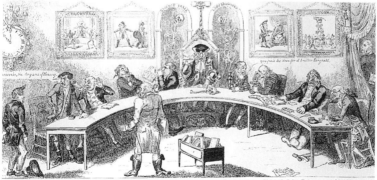

The EXAMINATION of a YOUNG SURGEON.

Fig. 24.1

examiners think and what they are looking for, and by not wasting time studying the same thing in three or four different ways.

Sadly most students give no thought contemplating any of these and rush away in search of medico-babble which they hope will give the impression of fathomless depths of erudition, judgement and wisdom.

How to study

Know your examination; reconnoitre the ground if you must treat it as war. A printed syllabus takes the place of a battle map, giving some indication of the campaign. Talking to successful candidates can be useful; talking to failed candidates is less useful; talking to an examiner will give the view of the other side of the table and need not be regarded as crawling.

The art of study is to recognize what is essential and what is decoration and not to waste time studying the same subject in several different ways in several different books because their fundamental similarity is obscured by slight variations of emphasis and major variations of language.

As an example taken from my own student days, psychiatrists taught us how to diagnose schizophrenia and, during the same term, a police surgeon taught us how to decide if a motorist had consumed more alcohol than was strictly safe. The essence of both was to demonstrate dislocation from reality – in one case, because of psychosis and in the other because of intoxication. The whole of medicine and its related subjects are shot through with many such examples – apparently disconnected yet each capable of description as one set of principles with one set of words.

In the pre-clinical years, each time the instruction manual dissected its way to a new anatomical region – from the axilla to the hand, from the abdomen to the feet – it uncovered peripheral nerves snaking between the muscles. Each time one was named, so was its inevitable spray of branches to skin, follicles, blood vessels and so on and students then had to learn several times something that required learning only once.

These branches are the same, whether they sprout from the ulnar nerve or the sciatic nerve and the major portion of a distinguished answer in regional anatomy can be constructed from them before any mention has to be made of where they actually are.

If picking up the thread that links essentials is the first step, then the second is to form an opinion about them – all of them;

this fixes them in the mind as golden nuggets of genuine knowledge, the glitter of which sheds light on any dark gaps uncovered in between them by hard questioning.

This habit of reasoning around fundamentals, polished in practice, hardens into a gleaming surface that will not crack in the white heat of an examination.

The study of all clinical subjects can be as ordered as the study of anatomy. Although the details may change we need frameworks which are unchanging, and indeed which belong to all branches of medicine. Any clinical subject can be studied and answered on the basis of four cardinal elements:

1. pathology
2. essential symptoms
3. essential signs
4. essential management.

1. We know that the eye is an organ of limited response. We also know that, should the condition in question produce some remote complication, there is a fair chance that it will involve the aqueous dynamics and the intraocular pressure. It cannot be difficult to find parallels between this and any other branch of medicine we care to mention.

2. There are but five essential symptoms and we can work out from the processes of pathology which of these symptoms might be triggered and why.

3. The essential signs do not change from condition to condition although decades of ophthalmic teaching would have us believe that they do.

4. Essential management is the same, no matter what part of the body is involved. We have to:

a. diagnose and find the cause
b. eliminate the cause if we can
c. deal with the effects of the cause (complications)
d. relieve pain
e. restore function.

All this can be attempted by medical means or surgical means – first of all in the short term and secondly in the long term.

The preceding framework must be in position before the examination, in the subconscious mind at the brain-stem level, releasing the conscious mind to observe, reason and respond at speed in the certainty that nothing has been missed.

WRITTEN PAPERS

The prime aim in any examination is to persuade the examiners that you have an ordered mind, that you grasp your subject and that you do not pad out your answers with question-begging, special pleading and needless repetition.

Even less convincing is the answer, for which an hour was allowed, scribbled over half a page, with the postscript 'time' – somehow meant to suggest a brain so teeming with information that an hour was not long enough to allow the candidate to decide what should be left out.

The written examination is the ideal opportunity, to notch up extra marks at leisure, because there is no face-to-face contact with an examiner whom the candidate might perceive as awesome.

The injunction not to study twice what needs to be studied only once applies equally to the construction of written answers. Every statement of consequence should be defended. An examiner will not be impressed by an inventory of capital words, stressing that the management of some disorder or another is important because it is serious, because it is vital, because it is critical. These are simply repetitions of something not yet proven.

The treatment of iritis is not 'steroids, four times a day'. This level of answer simply will not do. We have to define the problem – inflammation of the iris, which if untreated may lead on to

1. a secondary rise of pressure
2. adhesions between the iris and the lens
3. destruction of the eye
4. cataract
5. spontaneous resolution.

The treatment, slotting into its place in the framework of management in general is then the suppression of that inflammation with topical corticosteroids because, if it is not suppressed, then these possible complications might follow. That said, there is then no need to keep reminding the examiner that the inflammation has to be suppressed.

We should now be in a position to construct an answer on, say, herpes zoster ophthalmicus – the aetiology, pathology, clinical features, complications and management. This may sound alarming, but it is absolutely founded on simple principles and might read as follows:

ANSWER

Space demands that this be constructed in note form. However, in the examination, a major answer should be constructed as an essay, which of course implies the use of sentences and some attempt at literary composition.

The **diagnosis** is made from the classical distribution of the vesicles.

Management

Problems

1. Dermatitis. Infection of the broken vesicles. Scar formation. Late intractable pain.
2. Conjunctivitis. Pain. Secondary infection.
3. Keratitis
   Acute. Loss of vision due to superficial punctate keratitis.
   Chronic. Corneal scars if the active lesions penetrate Bowman's membrane.
   Cornea vulnerable because of virus-induced anaesthesia.
4. Iritis.
   Acute. Pain. Loss of vision. Floaters.
   Chronic. Adhesions. Iris to the lens. Secondary glaucoma. Damage to the trabecular meshwork. Secondary rise in pressure, cataract.

Treatment

1. Dermatitis

Short term: The aim is to kill the virus and to allow bacteria-free healing with minimal scar formation.

Acyclovir skin cream five times daily deals with the first problem. Thereafter an application which combines an antibiotic with corticosteroid may achieve both these aims to some degree. Their dosage will depend on the severity of the condition.

Long term: The pain of shingles is devastating and long term analgesics and emotional support may still not be enough to prevent thoughts of suicide.

2. Conjunctivitis

The aim is to prevent secondary infection from spreading to the cornea.

The application of topical antibiotics in a dose related to the severity usually achieves the above aims.

3. The cornea

Short term: Breach of corneal epithelium. The aim is to persuade the epithelium to heal. This is one condition where the danger of topical corticosteroids in the presence of a broken corneal epithelium is outweighed by their benefit in suppressing inflammation. But sometimes circumstances have to be created to allow the cornea to heal in its own time.

Closure of the eyelids with adhesive tape is ideal, but may not be easy because the broken skin on the eyelids might prevent the tape from sticking, whilst severe iritis requires constant topical treatment.

Frequent application of artificial tears goes some way to making the cornea feel that the eyelids are closed, which is its ideal state, even in health.

Long term: An anaesthetic cornea is a vulnerable cornea, and years after the acute attack this may lead to recurrent breakdown of the corneal epithelium.

Tape closure is by far the best way to give the cornea the circumstances it likes best.

When the cornea has recovered, it may be kept that way by closing the eyelids from time to time (perhaps one weekend out of three) on a regular basis. There is no precise time scale.

4. Iritis

The aim is to suppress inflammation and prevent complications in the acute phase.

Complications and restoration of function dominate the management of the chronic phase.

Short term: Topical corticosteroids – the dose is related to the severity of the inflammation.

Mydriatics – if the pupil shows signs of adhering to the lens, then dilating it will make the development of adhesions less likely to be complete.

If the intraocular pressure be raised, then it must be brought down.

Acetazolamide reduces the production of aqueous. However, it also produces systemic effects in the form of increased diuresis, finger tingling, kidney stones, metabolic acidosis and possibly even mental upset.

Topical beta-blockers – these drugs also reduce the production of aqueous, but with fewer side effects in most patients. However, they can delay the healing of corneal epithelium, and indeed may cause an intact epithelium to break down.

Long term: The intraocular pressure may remain permanently raised and will therefore require long-term treatment, possibly with beta-blockers or other anti-glaucoma drugs, or even drainage surgery. This is the age of chronic simple glaucoma and we must be sure that the condition we are dealing with really is secondary.

Cataract: There should be no particular complication in the removal of cataract. It is always best to restore the lost focus with an intraocular lens, but if there are problems in controlling intrao-

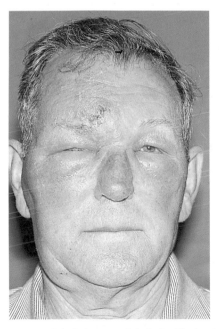

Fig. 24.2 Herpes zoster ophthalmicus – ophthalmic shingles due to infection along the first division of the trigeminal nerve. With the advent of acyclovir, the full-blown florid picture is becoming a rarity.

cular pressure before surgery, these may be worse after surgery, and may indeed require further surgery to control them.

Treatment before disease is established. The best management of all would be to abort all complications before they come into being. This can sometimes be achieved by systemic acyclovir if we can catch the disease in its prodromal phase.

The flaw in this approach is that we must catch the condition almost before we know what it is. People tend to put up with pain in the forehead; it is only the appearance of vesicles and worse that persuade them to seek attention.

Acyclovir tablets are expensive. The dosage is four times the standard – 800 mg five times daily for 7 days. But treating the complications in their full flower is probably more expensive still, not to mention the price in continued misery.

The pedestrian simplicity of this answer must come as a disappointment to all those who are seeking the passport to that rarified wonderland – that Arcania where the most unlikely conditions are diagnosed by guesswork, then confirmed by the most uncommon investigations and then treated by the most radical stratagems imaginable – clearly a land where canaries dare and where no sparrows fly.

ORAL EXAMINATIONS

Ideally these meetings should be conducted as conversations between equals, and if they are not, the fault almost invariably lies with the candidate.

The quality of response is measured by order, grasp of fundamentals and the very sensible realization that the examiner is looking for large-print principles and not a word-for-word repetition of page 2000 from whatever textbook happens to be the fashion of the year.

Any human meeting is an interplay of personality quirks, frailties and deeply held convictions. It is not the examiners alone who have a monopoly of personality flaws. At least, examination bodies try to root them out on their side of the table. However, they have no power to do the same thing for the candidates. The total elimination of human oddities would be impossible because indeed they are the warp and weft of life. In any case, after the examination – and there is life after the examination – successful candidates will encounter eccentricities far worse than anything conjured up at a Royal College of this or that.

CANDIDATES

Apart from frank ignorance, which may be the result of opening too many rather than too few textbooks, candidates regularly fail examinations for the following reasons:

1. They have no ordered framework for study.
2. They have formed no opinions of their own.
3. They waste time discovering the pet subjects of local examiners hoping to greet each with an inventory of their favourite beliefs. That they may have been misinformed or that it was all worthless information anyway never seems to put an end to this traffic in misguided faith.
4. Their brains are top-heavy with small-print minutiae at the expense of large-print essentials.
5. They fancy that they and the examiner have memorized the same book and that success must come mechanically if they can only identify which page the examiner has in mind, whereupon the pair of them can sit back to enjoy a shared memory.

Examiners do not memorize textbooks and they certainly do not read them up for the examination. Candidates, particularly those for whom English is not their native tongue, would spare themselves much unhappiness if they grasped this fact now, because if they do not, they will find themselves not only not enjoying a shared memory but perhaps being told that although the memory may be right, the content is wrong.

Most candidates believe that the examiner will be impressed if they can discharge all their detailed knowledge immediately, preferably in one sentence. Even if the torrent of information were intelligible it leaves the candidate nothing to decorate bare principles with later. No examiner will ever quibble with a general statement first. In fact they invariably prefer answers given that way.

So a question on the principles of applanation tonometry should not release an instant flood of detail about the formula for the area of a circle, the constituents of the ideal fluorescein anaesthetic mixture, a disquisition on surface tension and on the dangers of infection.

The opening statement must surely be that applanation tonometry is a way of measuring intraocular pressure; that a flat surface is applied to a curved surface at an increasing pressure. When the area of contact flattens, the pressure within equals the pressure without. That may well be enough. If details are asked then the questions will guide the candidate into which details are needed.

A good working rule is that we should always ask ourselves first, is there some prefatory statement that should have been made before the statement that is actually being made – some peg of first principles on which to hang later details?

Someone is bound to be asked about Horner's syndrome, and is equally likely to release a breathless list of causes, involving fractures of the cervical vertebra, tabes dorsalis, syringomyelia, apical tuberculosis and so on. The syndrome may indeed be caused by all of these things but that does not give any clue to the examiner that this is not just simply a list memorized from a huge textbook.

We could be tempted to say that Horner's syndrome is caused by paralysis of the cervical sympathetic nervous system, but it is possible that we should take one step further back still and describe it as an affection of one eye characterized by ptosis and miosis – because that is the first thing we see. The next statement could implicate the cervical sympathetic and thereafter, if asked, the more common causes could be considered.

The concept of syndromes is not encouraged in this book but medicine would not be medicine without a bit of tradition. The syndromes of tradition should at least form familiar patterns, but what should be the response to questions about a 30-year-old with sudden onset of horizontal diplopia?

The answer is not a salvo of pathology from demyelination to an intracranial aneurysm – though one of them may be to blame. We must first define the problem and break it up into categories. Is the diplopia monocular or binocular? If binocular, is it a latent squint breaking down, a frank paralysis of an extraocular muscle, or is the latter masquerading as the former? Each category is then open for discussion and wise candidates can direct that discussion to where they feel most comfortable.

The greatest source of disquiet to an examiner is the candidate who does not answer the question but sits paralysed in a long and terrible silence. This absence of speech can be quite as destructive as the gush of detail. The most likely cause is an instinctive assumption that the answer must be in detail, and no detail comes to mind. The answer, dare we repeat it again, should be in principle and no candidate should approach an examination bereft of basic principles.

For those whose mother tongue is not English, it is as well to learn several ways of phrasing the same idea well in advance of the examination. It makes things needlessly difficult if, in addition to the subject under scrutiny, the connecting phrases have to be continually translated into an unfamiliar tongue.

These phrases should be constructed for multiple use, ready to be deployed for strange subjects, unexpected subjects and examiners who appear to be beyond pleasing. If the linguistic translations are prepared in advance, then the conscious mind is free for the imaginative leaps necessary to keep the oral examination ticking along.

We have also to recognize that candidates meet not only examiners, they also meet other candidates who all appear to have been asked terribly clever questions to which they knew all the terribly clever answers on matters unfamiliar to everyone else. The rule is to note that, at the end of the examination, those with the loudest mouths and the cleverest answers are almost invariably absent from the list when the successful candidates are posted.

Hopeful examinees often add to their own sense of anguish with last-minute study. One such has been observed reading Gray's anatomy whilst attempting to deal with last-minute spasms of the bladder. Whatever else he passed, it was not the anatomy examination, although some allowance should have been made for manual and cerebral dexterity.

EXAMINERS

Examiners do not all come out of the same box. The ideal examiner will try to put candidates at their ease and ask one or two personal questions that moisten the tongue and allow it to separate from the palate. Not every examiner, however, is ideal and we have all come across exceptions from time to time. It is important to recognize that, apart from the very odd exception, most examiners think that they are good examiners and are certain that they are motivated by the highest principles. We are all victims of our own self-perception but, if candidates are going to be courtiers, they have to remember that all kings are more or less beautiful. As candidates, therefore, we have to recognize that examiners are in the driving seat and that nothing is to be gained by impertinence, arrogance or dishonesty.

The furrowed brow

Such displays of anguish may have nothing to do with our answers but with the examiner's concern that justice be done. But when every answer is met with a grimace worse than the one before, we might feel in the circumstances that it is we who are responsible. It could well be reasonable then to try to find out if we are disturbing the examiner in some way – asking if the answer was the sort of response that was wanted.

The single answer

Not infrequently a question may be asked with a single answer in mind when there may well be ten other answers, all equally correct. We have all been through it: working our way through an inventory of replies whilst the examiner keeps shaking the head and saying 'But is there not something else?'

If we appear to be getting nowhere near the magic answer and our confidence is collapsing, the way out is to persuade the examiner to recognize that the other answers were all relevant. A straight question as to their relevance might be the simplest stratagem.

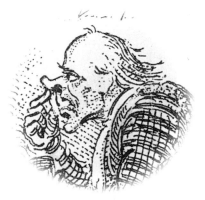

Fig. 24.3

A variation on the single answer

This might appear at first to be another version of the last example but it is not. Sometimes examiners might ask candidates to perform a small manoeuvre like tying a surgical knot. Although the term surgical knot is used glibly and frequently, there is no such thing as a surgical knot. The candidate may well realize this and not quite know how to respond when a piece of string is placed on the table.

In these circumstances we take refuge again in first principles. We might answer that knots in surgery (note the use of the words 'surgery' and 'knot' but with the order reversed) will vary in different circumstances and with different suture materials.

The essence of a knot is that it should fulfil its purpose. It should be unobtrusive; it should not slip. The 'sliding granny knot' of retinal surgery would not be suitable for a corneal graft because the surgical needs and the material are different.

That said, there is then no reason why the candidate cannot then tie whatever knot the examiner requests.

The angry examiner

Anger is unforgivable but it does happen from time to time at the end of a long trying day of orals, and it may be brought on by a candidate apparently dodging the issue or avoiding the point or not answering the question asked or simply sitting in silence.

Obviously it is in our interests to understand why the examiner has become irate, if we can and if we have enough conscious mind available to deal with the added pressure. It is at this point that the wisdom of prepared phrases becomes evident.

The first essential is to keep cool, which means counting to three, breathing deeply the while and not bursting into tears. This might well have worked with Napoleon, whom tears generally reduced to impatient blotting paper, but the average male examiner would simply wait for the storm to pass and the average female examiner would probably not wait at all.

Should the anger become intolerable, then it is perfectly reasonable to ask the examiner what we have done to produce such rage – and the phrases we use must of course be tried out and practised before venturing them in the white heat of an examination.

It is helpful sometimes to remind the examiner that we have had a teacher possibly not unlike the person in front of us at the moment and that our whole approach has been taught to us by someone and not just acquired unaided from a textbook.

Expected answer wrong

It has not been unknown for candidates to be asked their opinion of light flashing. We all know that light flashing can have a basis in the retina or in the optic pathways – as far back as the cerebral cortex. If the examiner were to interrupt an answer explaining all this by saying 'no' and that light flashing was caused by retinal detachment, then it is absolutely critical to stick to our point without causing offence.

We might say that we understood that light flashing was due to traction on the retina and that when the retina had torn the light flashing stopped. We might then ask the examiner 'is this not the case?'. If we can then persuade the examiner to join in the discussion, that in fact it might be so, then we have brought things back to the level of discussion and not the realm of machine-gun answering.

When I was a lad

Time catches up with all of us and examiners who have always perceived themselves as young and forward-looking may not have realized that they have become old and backward looking. 'When I was a lad' is a coded message favouring an old technique that may indeed be no longer be in use.

Clearly, to say that something is out of date is not wise, particularly if the examiner has fond memories of it. It would, however, be perfectly acceptable to emphasize that our teachers have told us something quite different because of some perfectly valid reason. If this answer can be given in a way that implies that the only real difference is youth and inexperience, then there can be no reason for the examiner to take umbrage.

Examiner with a story

A candidate was once told by the examiner, 'I was at my golf club last night and I woke up blind. What do you think might be wrong?'

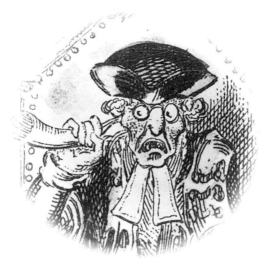

Fig. 24.4

It would be easy to imagine ourselves adrift in the quicksands of unreality, expected to provide a diagnosis on half a story and no signs. Most candidates who come to grief do so because they believe that this is the question.

It is not the question. We are being asked not to make a diagnosis immediately but to explain how we would arrive at our diagnosis.

Henry Longhurst used to say that putting was easy once emotion was removed from it. The same goes for the examination. All we need do is reason as we would in our own clinic, except this time in front of an audience. The diagnostic wheels should by now be revolving around:

1. possible causation
2. symptoms that might belong to the different causes
3. signs that would indicate one or other of the likely causes.

Pathology

Conceivable causes of visual loss in a middle-aged man – presumably reasonably fit. If the examiner is portly and florid and breathing with difficulty, that might add a cause or two to our list but of course diplomacy will dictate how far these additions should be put into words.

Symptoms

We must never say 'I would take a good history'. What other history would we take? What we have to say is that we would want to know from the history what the patient meant by blindness. We would have to edit the history and ask questions directed towards whichever of the possible causes we have in mind. Is there total loss of light perception? If not, how much is left? Has it ever happened before? Had anything been consumed in large quantities? – after all it was a golf club and not a church social.

The seven signs

By this time we should, on automatic pilot, have arrived at the conclusion that the reason for bilateral visual reduction to the level of light perception is most likely to be found somewhere in the optic nerves. If the golf club were an essential part of the story and not merely interpolated to add verisimilitude, then the most likely explanation would be a job lot of methanol passed off to the club as whisky.

But suppose the examiner is looking for the single answer of Eales disease, doubtless parrying every correct answer with 'and what else?'

This means the story was a genuine episode and not a fictional tale concocted for the examination. It has to be conceded that bilateral vitreal haemorrhage would not be the first on the list of conditions to explain bilateral blindness. It would therefore be absolutely acceptable to defend a diagnosis of bilateral optic neuritis with edited abstracts from the essential symptoms and from the essential signs.

The message here is loud and clear. It does not always matter if we come to the wrong conclusion, provided we come to it in the right way.

Experience

Occasionally, in a surgical oral, the examiner, in the face of some stumbling answer, might ask if the candidate has done this or that operation before. The answer may well be 'no', but that does not imply that the candidate must fail. The operation may be one that is not practised by every ophthalmologist but by those with a subspecialty.

The response must therefore be not just simply 'no', but 'no' and why. We might say that, where we have trained, this has been considered as a subspecialty operation to be done by an expert only. Thereafter, however, we should then be prepared to go on and discuss the technique. In other words we have not just delivered an unvarnished 'no'. By qualifying it, we have in fact turned our practical inexperience into the positive feature which in fact it is.

CLINICAL EXAMINATIONS

The clinical section of the examination proper is merely an extension of the golfer with the visual handicap and in no way parallels a normal out-patient clinic – but then that is the way of clinical examinations. It is a measure of our skill as a candidate to turn these artificial anomalies of the examination into something that we do every day.

We will almost invariably be asked to do the one thing that this book emphasizes that we should not do – namely to look at a fundus and make a decision without any information from the essential symptoms or the seven signs. We can appear the thoughtful clinicians we really are by recognizing what aspects of real life are missing and by arriving at our diagnosis by the landmarks described above.

Coming to a sensible clinical conclusion face-to-face, be it from a fundal appearance or from a story, calls above all things for a clear, ordered technique, which is as follows:

The eye, dare we repeat it, is an organ or limited response. We must regard each of these responses as a terminus to which lines run from different pathological starting points. Along these lines stops can be made at the essential symptoms and the seven signs. Which of the symptoms and signs we stop at will be determined by the starting point and the terminus. Stopping at them all would clearly take a long time, would certainly irritate the examiner and might end up arriving at the wrong terminus anyway. The secret, as ever, is to edit.

Presented with a terminus (a fundal appearance) we can edit our way back to a starting point. Presented with a starting point we can edit our way down to a terminus.

When it comes to management, we have to remember that **there is no one answer in clinical medicine**.

Clinical responses are complexes of the perceived pathology, the particular needs of the particular patient, the particular views of a clinician, together with experience, past thinking and current thinking on the subject. The examiner doesn't want us to agree for the sake of agreement. What they want to know are our views on the matter, particularly in relation to our experience and why we would undertake such an approach. They want to know, in other words, if we are safe.

If we are left, then, with a fundal appearance, we should always remember that looking at the fundus, particularly with the direct ophthalmoscope, all that will come into view (if anything, indeed) will be the disc, the macula and the vessels. We should form an opinion on these and store that opinion. We should then see if there is any other feature that springs out and, when being asked about it, describe it as the dominant feature. If the examiner then asks 'What about the disc, the macula, the vessels?' then the reflex assimilation of their appearance would be there ready to describe.

It is vital to remember that the management of anything anywhere is to:

1. find the cause if we can
2. eliminate the causes if we can
3. deal with the complications
4. relieve pain
5. restore function.

   Each of these will be weighted differently

   — from medical to surgical
   — from short term to long term
   — from patient to patient
   — from circumstance to circumstance.

But the foundation of successful management is first to define what has to be managed. A binocular grandfather and a monocular boy may both have identical cataracts – but they cannot have identical indications for intervention.

That, then, is the secret of studying, sitting, passing and possibly even enjoying examinations. Although it may not appear obvious, the examiner is not looking to fail but to pass a candidate. It is a great sense of relief and indeed a pleasure when the candidate turns the examination into a discussion between equals. If candidates would only grasp this fact, and exchange a shaky knowledge of small print for a secure knowledge of large print, then there would be fewer drawn and anxious faces on examination day on either side of the table.

25. Epilogue

The constant message of this book is a rondo on three simple themes:

1. The eye is an organ of limited response.
2. The secret is to recognize a response and work out the cause later.
3. The patient's choice of the five symptoms and our unswerving application of the seven signs will tell us what we expect to see with the eighth sign – in the fundus.

When we find it, we can deal with it according to the timeless principles of management of any disease in any organ:

1. find the cause
2. eliminate the cause
3. eliminate the effects of the cause
4. relieve pain
5. restore function.

All of these are delivered by medical means or surgical means in the short term and in the long term.

Finally, if the seven signs draw a blank as to what is actually wrong, they will tell us unequivocally what is not wrong and that our patient has a safe eye. A safe eye is one that will not go blind because we have missed the things that people do not complain about:

1. creeping field loss
2. shallow anterior chamber
3. raised intraocular pressure.

All this can be summed up as observation along a pre-arranged framework, leaving the conscious mind free to speculate on the information that reaches us through our systematic survey.

A detective famous for his deerstalker, fiddle and tobacco stored in a Persian slipper made his name synonymous with this technique. His findings were a product of observation and reason and by the systematic elimination of causes that were not possible. His creator, Conan Doyle, based this aspect of his character on Joseph Bell, a former president of the Royal College of Surgeons of Edinburgh, whose uncanny deductions from the observation of apparently nothing were legendary. Even more momentous from our point of view, as a doctor Conan Doyle specialized in diseases of the eye.

A miscellany of words and drugs

accommodation – mechanism by which the eye changes focus, essentially from distance to near. Contraction of the ciliary muscle alters the shape of the lens. The act of accommodation produces constriction of the pupil.

acyclovir – has eclipsed idoxuridine in the treatment of herpes simplex infections. It has now been extended to the treatment of AIDS and has transformed the management of herpes zoster.

adrenaline – *see* **mydriatics**

agnosia – failure to recognize familiar objects despite intact vision.

antibacterials – topical applications customary for ocular infection. Chloramphenicol, framycetin, gentamicin and neomycin have a particularly wide spectrum. Gentamicin and tobramycin are used selectively to deal with *Pseudomonas aeruginosa*. Fusidic acid is of particular use in staphylococcal infections.

amaurosis fugax – The 'g' is usually pronounced as a 'j', against all rules of English. It means transient visual loss either of one eye or one field.

amblyopia – formal term for a lazy eye. The central vision is diminished or lost in an eye with otherwise no demonstrable physical defect.

aniridia – congenital absence of the iris.

aniseikonia – each eye perceives visual perceptions of the same object as different in size. An obstacle to binocular vision.

anisometropia – another obstacle to binocular vision. It results from a discrepancy between the refractive needs of each eye. Uncorrected or uncorrectable, it can result in amblyopia (laziness) of the eye with the greater refractive error.

anophthalmos – the extremely rare absence of a genuine eyeball.

anterior chamber – space bounded in front by the cornea, behind by the iris and filled with aqueous fluid that enters through the pupil and leaves through the trabecular meshwork in the angle.

aphakia – absence of the natural lens.

aphasia – a synonym for dysphasia: may be receptive or expressive and usually a combination of both. The expressive type is essentially a disorder in language construction but not of comprehension, giving rise to extreme and wholly understandable distress. Receptive dysphasia is a disorder of language analysis. An affected individual can neither appreciate nor act upon instructions. Location of the cause is not always easy but receptive dysphasia incriminates the dominant tempero-parietal lobe. Expressive dysphasia, on the other hand, must incriminate the motor cortex.

aqueous – clear salt solution that fills the anterior chamber and provides a blood substitute for the transparent tissues – cornea, lens and vitreous.

astigmatism – error of refraction which prevents light from coming to a point focus on the retina because the eye is optically oval.

atropine sulphate *see* **cycloplegics**

beta-blockers – beta-adrenoreceptor-blocking agents are now the sheet anchor in the treatment of raised intraocular pressure. They reduce the inflow and increase the outflow. May produce deposits on contact lenses to the point where they are mutually exclusive. All beta-blockers slow the heart and may precipitate cardiac failure. Some may cause asthma and the lipid-soluble variety can effect the brain, bringing about hallucinations and disturbance of sleep. Although timolol and carteolol are more effective in absolute reduction of intra-ocular pressure, there is some evidence that betaxolol preserves the visual field for longer.

binocular vision – capacity of the eyes to work together, focusing and fusing images viewed from slightly different angles into one three-dimensional image.

blepharitis – inflammation of the skin of the eyelids. There is usually scaling around the lash margin, producing a sort of eyelid dandruff. A destructive ulcerative form is very rare.

buphthalmos – now taken as synonymous with infantile glaucoma. The enlarged eyeball with its stretched sclera resembling that of an ox is thought to be the result of raised intraocular pressure in infancy.

canaliculi – drainage ducts for tears in the upper and lower eyelids connecting the lacrimal puncta with the common canaliculus, which itself enters the lacrimal sac.

canthus – name given to the angle where the upper lid joins the lower lid.

carbonic anhydrase inhibitors – the original diuretics, the most celebrated of which is acetazolamide. They reduce aqueous production but in the long term have certain side effects. Acetazolamide has now been recast in a new formulation, allowing a much more even release of the drug than has hitherto been possible. There is some evidence that the systemic malaise previously ascribed to the drug itself has actually been caused by uneven absorption.

cataract – any opacification of the natural lens.

chalazion – the quiescent end-result of inflammation of one of the tarsal glands.

chloramphenicol – most popular topical broad-spectrum antibacterial agent. It retains its efficacy best when stored in a refrigerator. Rare reports of aplastic anaemia through systemic absorption of eye drops cannot be regarded as a serious contraindication to its use.

choroid – posterior section of the uveal tract providing the red reflex visible to the ophthalmoscope through the transparent retina.

chloroquine – widely used in the management of certain collagen disorders such as systemic lupus erythematosus and rheumatoid arthritis and as a prophylaxis against malaria. White subepithelial corneal deposits have been described in some 30% of patients on long-term treatment. Disturbance of the retinal pigment epithelium can result in central loss and constriction of the peripheral fields. Up to 1 g a day in the short term is the accepted safe level, but there is a cumulative effect in the long term.

ciliary body – middle portion of the uveal tract connecting the iris to the choroid. The natural lens is suspended from the ciliary processes. The ciliary muscle is the muscle of accommodation. The ciliary epithelium, providing the aqueous fluid, is the heart of the eye.

coloboma – persistence of primitive vascular tissue together with failure of fusion of the developing optic vessel results in a congenital cleft of varying dimensions in the lower nasal quadrant. It may range from a slight notch in the eyelid to a complete gap in the uveal tract all the way back to the optic nerve head.

colour vision (and defects) – the eye perceives light between 400 and 700 nm and perceives colour with its colour receptors. Each cone has a maximal perception of red, green or blue. Ocular perception depends on the nature of ambient light. It is customary to describe colour in terms of hue, brightness and saturation. The *hue* depends on reflection, radiation or transmission of light of particular wave lengths. Shading is brought about by the addition of black. *Brightness* is related to light intensity. *Saturation* indicates the purity of a particular hue. Colour blindness is usually inherited as an X-linked characteristic and, apart from exclusion from certain occupations, should not cause any serious visual disturbance.

conjunctiva – wet membrane formed in loose folds between the eyelid and the eyeball. It is like the synovial sac of a ball and socket joint.

convergence – act of pulling the visual axes out of parallel for near vision.

cornea – transparent anterior wall of the eye continues with the sclera and the anterior limit of the anterior chamber.

corticosteroids – The cause of many complications, both short- and long-term: they can catastrophically accelerate the corneal destruction in herpes simplex keratitis; they may raise the intra-ocular pressure in sensitive individuals (steroid responders) and induce posterior sub-capsular cataract. Recently there is some evidence to suggest that oral corticosteroids given in the hope of cutting short an attack of demyelinating optic neuritis may make a second attack more likely.

crystalline lens – the convex focusing device suspended from the ciliary processes separating the vitreal cavity from the anterior chamber. The term 'crystalline' is going out of fashion.

cycloplegics – drugs that paralyse the ciliary muscle and accommodation, resulting in a dilated pupil and failure of near vision. Atropine is the most famous and long-acting but is now used only in the treatment of iritis. Simple dilatation is brought about by cyclopentolate and, more recently, tropicamide, the action of which wears off in a morning. Adrenaline is not a cycloplegic. It stimulates the dilator pupillae directly.

cylindrical lens – used in the treatment of astigmatism, it focuses in one meridian only.

dacryocystitis – infection that sometimes ends in an abscess of the tear sac.

dark adaptation – capacity of the retina to increase its sensitivity in response to decreased illumination.

dioptre – unit by which the strength of lenses is measured.

diplopia – double vision. Monocular implies some opacity. Binocular indicates a paralysis of an extraocular muscle or imbalance of the eyes.

ectropion – separation between (usually) the lower lid and the eyeball. Hereditary in bloodhounds, the unfortunate result of passing time in the rest of us. In both circumstances the eyes become dry, exposed and inflamed.

endophthalmitis – gross intraocular inflammation, usually the result of infection.

enophthalmos – reverse of proptosis. The eyeball sinks into the orbit, either because of orbital fracture or because of spontaneous shrinkage of the globe itself.

entropion – reverse of ectropion. The eyelid turns inwards, abrading the cornea with the lashes.

enucleation – surgical removal of the eye.

epiphora – another term for watering.

'E' test – testing of visual acuity in those who for one reason or another cannot read.

Excimer laser – a method of sculpting the corneal curvature to reduce myopia and astigmatism.

exenteration – extirpation of the entire contents of the orbit down to the bone, usually for advanced intraorbital malignancy.

exophthalmos – another name for proptosis: the eyeball in advance of where it ought to be.

floaters – opacities, usually in the vitreous but sometimes in the anterior chamber, recognized by patients in their field of vision. Most floaters appear the same. It is their companions that determine their significance.

fovea – the absolute centre of the macula where the most exact detail is noted.

fundus – the interior of the eye as seen with the ophthalmoscope.

fusidic acid – broad spectrum antibiotic most effective against staphylococci. *Viscous drops do not blur vision whilst remaining active on a twice-daily basis.*

gentamicin – broad-spectrum antibiotic drops or ointment form.

glaucoma – the most precise meaning is an optic neuropathy characterized by particular field defects and disc cupping and usually related to raised intraocular pressure. It also is taken to mean the named disease chronic simple glaucoma. The confusion is compounded by five other meanings: acute glaucoma (angle closure); any rise of intraocular pressure be the cause known or not; any rise of intraocular pressure where the cause is identified (secondary glaucoma); buphthalmos – infantile glaucoma. It would make most sense to reserve the name for the pathological process and describe everything else as a raised intraocular pressure.

guttae – Latin plural of 'gutta' meaning drop. Precedes name of drug prescribed in drop form, e.g. Guttae (G.) Chloramphenicol.

hemianopia – field loss related to one side of the body affecting both eyes through their cerebral connection to the other side of the body.

hippus – although the name might imply some large muscular animal, it refers to small muscular movements in the iris – fine rhythmic minute dilatation and constriction. It is of no consequence.

hordeolum – commonly known as a stye. It is indeed much less common than infected tarsal cyst.

hypermetropia (long sight) – error of refraction which forces the eye to focus as for reading when it is seeing in the distance. Even the young eye may have used up all its reading focus when it actually tries to see for near.

intrinsic sympathomimetic activity (ISA) – certain compounds both antagonize and stimulate adrenergic receptors. In theory at least, they are less likely to cause bradycardia and coldness of the extremities.

Ishihara plates – colour test for red–green colour defects. Operated by asking patients to recognize numbers, trace lines and recognize jumbles against a series of multicoloured dots.

keratoconus – deformity where the natural dome shape of the cornea gives way to that of a cone.

laser – acronym from Light Amplification by Stimulated Emission of Radiation. An artificial method of selecting a wavelength of light which may then be directed with great accuracy to any spot within the eye. As the wavelength moves towards the red end of the spectrum its absorption moves deeper through the pigment epithelium into the choroid. *Not* the treatment of choice for retinal detachment.

limbus – margin between the sclera and the cornea. Limbal injection, or certain corneal injection, is the deep redness indicating one of the three serious red eyes.

macula – posterior pole temporal to the optic nerve head centred on the fovea – the acute area of central vision.

microphthalmos – congenital defect resulting in a tiny and usually useless eyeball.

miotics – drugs which produce constriction of the pupil. They may also drag on the peripheral retina. The only one now used in ophthalmology is pilocarpine.

mydratics – drugs which cause dilatation of the pupil with or without paralysing the ciliary muscle. Adrenaline or its pro-drug dipivefrin or phenylephrine produce mydriasis by stimulation of the sympathetic nervous system.

myopia (short sight) – error of refraction in which the eye cannot see in the distance. The distance focus is close to the eye and the near focus closer still.

non-steroidal anti-inflammatory agents – a topical drug which can suppress ocular inflammation as effectively as corticosteroids without raising the pressure, causing cataract or fostering infection has for years been a philosopher's stone for the pharmaceutical chemists. The most recent, diclofenac sodium, would appear to meet all these requirements more impressively than its predecessors.

nystagmus – rapid involuntary movement of the eye at any speed in any direction.

oculentum – Latin singular for ointment: precedes name of drug in ointment form, e.g. Oculentum (Oc.) Chloramphenicol.

photocoagulation – technique to produce a chorio-retinal scar by the absorption of light and its conversion to heat by the pigment epithelium.

presbyopia – refractive state of advancing years when the hardening lens no longer responds to the demands of the ciliary muscle.

proptosis – eyeball pushed forwards out of the orbit.

pterygium – overgrowth of episcleral and subconjunctival tissues which moves across the cornea, usually from the nasal limbus. Common in desert dwellers and sailors.

ptosis – drooping of the upper eyelid.

scotoma – an area within the visual field either partially sensitive or totally insensitive.

Snellen chart – the series of letters used to check the level of distance vision.

strabismus – squint.

sympathetic ophthalmitis – a pan-uveitis involving both eyes following a penetrating injury in one eye.

synechia – adhesion of the iris to anything within the anterior chamber.

uveal tract – iris, ciliary body and choroid, so named from its resemblance, through a thin sclera, to a black grape.

uveitis – one of the synonyms for inflammation of the uveal tract.

viscous drops – new formulation, at present restricted to fusidic acid but hopefully to be extended. Applied as an 'ointment', it becomes a drop, sustaining release of drug over a long period without blurring vision.

Index

Page numbers in **bold type** refer to illustrations.